Language Disorders in Children and Adults

Psycholinguistic Approaches to Therapy

Edited by

Shula Chiat, James Law and Jane Marshall
Department of Clinical Communication Studies
City University, London

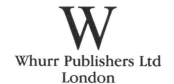

Whurr Publishers Ltd
London

© 1997 Whurr Publishers Ltd.
First published 1997 by
Whurr Publishers Ltd
19B Compton Terrace, London N1 2UN, England

British Library Cataloguing-in-Publication Data
A catalogue record for this book is available from the
British Library.

ISBN 1 86156 014 1

Printed and bound in the UK by Athenaeum Press Ltd,
Gateshead, Tyne & Wear

Contents

Acknowledgements

We would like to acknowledge the role played by Norma Corkish Director of AFASIC, and Ruth Coles from Action for Dysphasic Adults in setting up this collaborative venture.

We would like to thank the panel who contributed so much to the discussion of the papers at the conference:

Maria Black, University College London
Paul Fletcher, Hong Kong University
Sue Franklin, University of York
Joy Stackhouse, University College London

Contributors

Wendy Best is a researcher in the Department of Psychology, Birkbeck College, London and a speech and language therapist working with secondary school children with specific language problems

Maria Black is a lecturer in linguistics in the Department of Phonetics and Linguistics, University College London

Carolyn Bruce is a speech and language therapist, a researcher and a lecturer in the Department of Human Communication Science, University College London

Alison Bryan is a speech and language therapist working with children with specific language difficulties in North Herts NHS Trust

Shula Chiat is a senior lecturer in linguistics in the Department of Clinical Communication Studies, City University, London

Claire Gatehouse is a speech and language therapist and lecturer in the Department of Human Communication Science, University College London

Amanda Hampshire is a speech and language therapist working with children with specific language difficulties in North Durham Community Health Care Trust

David Howard is a speech and language therapist and professor in the Department of Speech, University of Newcastle upon Tyne

James Law is a senior lecturer in child language and a speech and language therapist in the Department of Clinical Communication Studies, City University, London

Sadie Lewis is a speech and language therapist working with children with specific language difficulties in the Lifespan Healthcare NHS Trust, Cambridgeshire

Jane Marshall is a speech and language therapist and lecturer in the Department of Clinical Communication Studies, City University, London

Kay Mogford-Bevan is a speech and language therapist, a developmental psychologist and senior lecturer in speech in the Department of Speech, University of Newcastle upon Tyne

Julie Morris is a speech and language therapist at Ryhope Hospital, Sunderland and a researcher in the Department of Psychology, University of York

Susan Pethers is a speech and language therapist at Addenbrooke's Hospital, Cambridge

Jane Speake is a speech and language therapist working with children with specific language difficulties in the Lifespan Healthcare NHS Trust, Cambridgeshire

Maggie Vance is a lecturer in developmental speech and language disorders and a speech and language therapist in the Department of Human Communication Science, University College London

Rosemary Varley is a lecturer in language disorder and a speech and language therapist in the Department of Speech Science, University of Sheffield

General introduction
Making new connections:
in whose interests?

SHULA CHIAT

In this book, for the first time, clinicians working with language-impaired children meet clinicians working with language-impaired adults in order to talk about individual therapy cases. The meeting which takes place here on paper arose from a live encounter at a conference of the same title which took place in June 1996. This conference was itself born of new connections between two voluntary groups AFASIC, and Action for Dysphasic Adults, and clinicians and researchers from City University.

In our view, this bringing together of work with children and adults has come about as a result of major shifts in our assumptions about the nature of their difficulties and about the goals and methods of our intervention. These shifts have opened up the possibility that children and adults may share similar impairments in language processing – even though those impairments have different origins and occur at very different stages of life – and that each may shed light on the other. By bringing them together, we hope to stimulate new questions and new insights into the obstacles which can arise in language processing and the ways in which these can be tackled. The case studies which came out of this meeting are presented here not as models, but as a contribution to debate about intervention in specific language impairments. This debate is opened up and developed in editorial chapters which introduce and conclude each section of the book.

Of course, there are many issues that are not shared between children and adults. For example, we can assume that the impact of a language impairment on a person's family and social life will be quite different depending upon their stage in the life cycle. Such social and emotional dimensions of language impairment are clearly very important, and if they are not tackled in any depth in this book, this is only because the focus of the book lies elsewhere.

Given its focus, the book will be of particular interest to therapists working with specific language impairment in children and adults. It

1

will also be of relevance to psycholinguists and cognitive neuropsychologists exploring the nature of language impairment and the effects of intervention.

The orientation of the book

To set the scene for the following case studies, we need to clarify the theoretical shifts which have brought them together.

Psycholinguistics and acquired aphasia

One such shift is the development of psycholinguistics and cognitive neuropsychology, which has provided the impetus for much recent research and practice with aphasic patients. **Psycholinguistics** is concerned with the processes by which language is understood and produced. It seeks to identify the nature of the representations which are processed in going from sound to meaning and from meaning to sound, and the mechanisms by which those representations are recognised, stored and retrieved. From a psycholinguistic point of view, language impairment is viewed as a breakdown at some point in these processes. **Cognitive neuropsychology** is also concerned with the way in which information is processed, but with the focus on people whose processing is impaired following brain damage as opposed to normal language processing. Cognitive neuropsychology is interested in all forms of information processing, including but not confined to language. However, when their target is language impairment, the concerns of psycholinguistics and cognitive neuropsychology converge. Both generate models of language processing which specify the types of information which are represented mentally (often characterised by 'boxes'), and the connections between those representations (often characterised by 'arrows'). Both enable us to formulate hypotheses about the components of the model which have been damaged in cases of language impairment. Both seek evidence of **dissociations** in an individual's language processing such that one component in the model is damaged while another is spared. Particularly telling are double dissociations, where different individuals show reverse patterns of damaged and spared information processing. Such dissociations may in turn provide evidence of the way that information is organised and so lead to refinement of language-processing models.

Psycholinguistics and aphasia therapy

In the wake of psycholinguistic and cognitive neuropsychological approaches to assessment in acquired aphasia came questions about therapy. If the psycholinguistic breakdown could be identified, what implications would this have for intervention? One assumption might be that the implications are direct: once you have identified the source of the impairment in a person's processing, that is what you work on. But finding out the source of the problem is not the same as finding out how it can be overcome. This depends not just on how processing works or fails to work, but on how processing can be affected through intervention. Therapy has come to be seen as a theoretical issue in its own right. This recognition has extended aphasia research from investigating the nature of the blocks in an individual's language processing, to investigating how psycholinguistic tasks might affect those blocks. Traditionally, a psycholinguistic approach has often been seen in opposition to a 'functional' approach which concerned itself less with the processing origins of the problem and more with its consequences for communication. However, this divide was probably always artificial, as psycholinguistically based therapy generally aims to be functional, and functional therapy generally relies on the individual's processing capacity to fulfil functions.

Psycholinguistics and language impairment in children

The impact of psycholinguistic theory and methodology on assessment and then therapy in acquired aphasia was not matched in the developmental field. In the case of language-impaired children, language-focused work involved linguistic description of their language output and input, largely for comparison with normal language development (one exception, perhaps, being early psycholinguistic work on phonological disorder in children). This focus on linguistic description and comparison pre-empted investigation into the processes which lay behind the child's comprehension and production of language. Language-focused therapy was then driven by developmental norms rather than by the child's processing.

Another major shift giving rise to this book has been the recent surge of interest in extending psycholinguistic thinking to language-impaired children. This has in part been driven by psycholinguistically-based therapies with adults which strike a chord with 'child' therapists. The original impetus, however, is the recognition that if psycholinguistic questions are not posed in relation to children, this is not for want of such questions. If children have specific difficulties with language, those difficulties must arise at some point in their processing of the connections between sound and meaning. Psycholinguistic questions about the point of breakdown in input/output processing are as pertinent to developmental as acquired disorders. However, they have appeared to be impossibly complicated by what we might term the 'developmental dimension'.

In the case of language-impaired adults, it is assumed that they had full representations of the words and structures of their language prior to their stroke, and that these representations have become damaged or inaccessible following the stroke. Language-impaired children, on the other hand, are in the process of acquiring the representations of their language. We can still pose questions about which aspects of those representations they have and which they do not have, but we cannot automatically attribute any limitation we observe to their processing impairment, as we can with adults.Why not?

First, a limitation in a child's representation may be due to their stage of development rather than their impairment. Children who are developing normally do not acquire adult representations instantaneously. Their acquisition of word and sentence structure is gradual, following patterns which are themselves the focus of psycholinguistic research. If a language-impaired child lacks certain information about words or sentences, this could be normal for their stage of language development or even for their age. If we are investigating their processing impairment, the aim is to identify constraints over and above those which occur in the course of normal development.

The second complicating factor with language-impaired children is that difficulties in processing some aspect of linguistic representations may result in difficulties further down the processing line. The most obvious illustration of this possibility is provided by deaf children acquiring spoken language. Here, the obstacle is known to occur at the earliest stage of input processing, but will affect all subsequent stages of input/output processing to some degree. This will limit the child's access to all aspects of spoken language representations. A similar situation may arise for children who have difficulties at later stages of input/output processing. A child who has difficulties in processing phonology in input and in establishing the phonological representations of words is likely to have difficulties with connecting phonological representations to meanings. Hence, a problem with word semantics could arise from a prior problem with word phonology. Difficulties with semantics may, in turn, give rise to difficulties in connecting meanings to phonological representations in output. Hence, a problem in phonological output could arise from a prior problem with semantics.

These examples illustrate how processing difficulties may disrupt the child's development and organisation of full adult representations. But if the child's representations are different or are organised differently from the adult's, would we not expect them to break down differently? For example, if the child has a difficulty in speech processing, this might be expected to disrupt the development of phonological representations. In contrast, the adult who has already established phonological representations may preserve these in the face of speech processing difficulties. On the other hand, the adult's established phonological representations – or semantic representations for that matter – might be open to impairments which could not occur in a child who had not established such representations in the first place. This may mean that some patterns of impairment observed in an adult's representations may fail to turn up in observations of children. For example, we may encounter adults who process concrete words more effectively than abstract words, or vice versa. But we are unlikely to discover such differences in young children since their exposure to abstract vocabulary would anyway be limited. A flip side of the developmental dimension, then, is the possibility that adults may show processing impairments for which children will not be eligible.

The developmental factors we have identified undoubtedly complicate the psycholinguistic enterprise with children, and the contribution of models of adult language processing in that enterprise. But they do not preclude it.

One way of taking account of factors due to the normal developmental process is to compare the language-impaired child's representations with those of normally developing children of the same general 'language age' (language-matched children). In carrying out research, this may be feasible and appropriate. But in clinical practice, it may be neither. Another view, though, is that the developmental factor ceases to be an issue with children of 5 years and over. By this age, normally developing children have their language pretty well under their belts. When a child's language is unusual – regardless of whether it is construed as 'delayed' or 'deviant' – we can surely infer that this is due to particular difficulties in language processing rather than just the developmental process. It is striking that the extension of psycholinguistic thinking to children has involved children beyond the age when normal children are going through very rapid and individually variable development in all domains and when it is well-nigh impossible to separate out the strands. The youngest child in the following case studies is 5 years 10 months. Here, the developmental dimension need not be an issue.

The other complicating factor, the possible impact of one aspect of language processing on another in development, is one to explore rather than eliminate. It is integral to the psycholinguistic enterprise. Theories of language development, normal or impaired, must address interactions between different aspects of linguistic representations in the developmental process. Here we meet the possibility that work with language-impaired children may give a lead to work with adults. One of the surprises of the following case studies – but one in line with much current theory and research – is that different aspects of linguistic representations may be less compartmentalised in adult processing than was earlier assumed. Interactions between different levels of processing may be as much an issue for adult language processing, normal and impaired, as they have been recognised to be with children.

The impact of one level on another, whether in children or adults, is increasingly the focus of therapy with both. One level may have negative repercussions on another, but the converse may also be true. A strength at one level may be exploited to strengthen another level or provide indirect access to it. For example, strength in a child's semantics might be actively used to consolidate weak phonological representations associated with semantics. An adult's strength in orthographic representations might be exploited to access or bolster phonological representations. Thus, the sort of interactions highlighted in the developmental field play an important role not only in theories about language processing and its impairment, but in generating and pursuing hypotheses about intervention.

Psycholinguistics and pragmatics

This is not the only area where developmental research may make the running. The domain of pragmatics has long been a focus of research and intervention with children. With adults, the focus has tended to be on specfically linguistic skills to the exclusion of pragmatic factors, except perhaps in right hemisphere patients. Only recently has interest in pragmatics grown, with the emergence of, for example, **conversational analysis** in adults with aphasia. Here, then, is another shift in the field which has led children and adults, coming from different angles, to converge.

In this book, the child–adult encounter in pragmatics joins with another encounter: between pragmatics and psycholinguistics. Traditionally, pragmatic skills have been distinguished from general cognitive skills or specifically psycholinguistic skills. Pragmatic intervention, rather like 'functional' intervention, has been counterposed to language-focused intervention. Pragmatic skills involve the structure of interactions with other individuals in context, and the content and form of language appropriate to those interactions. Such skills rest on the ability to process information about the context and interlocutors, and the connection between these and structures of language. The type of information to be processed is distinct from the information required in processing the forms and structures of language, but it is information processing nonetheless. Where a child's or adult's pragmatic skills appear to be impaired, we can again pose questions about the source of that impairment in their processing of information, in this case, about other people and about context. The final shift in assumptions which has motivated this book is one which it initiates – the extension of psycholinguistic thinking to pragmatic difficulties. The discussion of cases in the book takes the first steps in this direction, opening the way to a rich area of exploration.

This psycholinguistic venture into pragmatics indicates how far intervention has moved beyond the polarisation between narrowly 'linguistic' and broadly 'functional' approaches. Psycholinguistically motivated therapy addresses the full range of processes involved in using language.

The structure of the book

This conception of intervention, which integrates pragmatics into psycholinguistics, and psycholinguistics into therapy, creates the bridge between children and adults. It provides us with a common perspective on anyone with an impairment in language processing. But it leads us to consider each individually, the object being to explore, with the patient, what particular deficits occur in information processing and how these may be influenced by intervention.

In each case, the starting point is a hunch about the focus of the individual's difficulties, based on initial observation of their language production and comprehension. Typical initial hunches might be that difficulties lie primarily in word phonology, or in sentence structure, or in use of words and sentences in context. These hunches lead to the selection of initial assessments, to explore the hypothesised difficulties in input and output. Such assessments might alter or refine the original hunch. Their outcome will form the basis for initial hunches about the goals and methods of intervention. Intervention and the patient's response to it may contribute fresh insights into the difficulties, which may in turn lead to development or revision of the therapy hypothesis. The emphasis in this approach is on interactions: between intact and impaired levels of language processing; between observations emerging from assessment and those emerging from therapy; between the patient and therapist. Therapy so conceived is dynamic, moving from initial hypotheses about the sort of intervention that will facilitate the patient's processing, according to the patient's response to that intervention.

This approach to intervention provides the rationale for the following presentation of case studies of therapy. Two are presented in each section, one child and one adult. Child and adult are paired on the basis of the therapist's initial hunch about the source of difficulty: whether it is in phonological, lexical, sentence, or pragmatic processing. Each pair of therapy studies is preceded by an introduction with examples of how difficulties in each of these areas may manifest themselves and an overview of the processing involved. The child and adult cases are then presented in turn, and followed by a discussion of similarities and differences between them. Though all the therapy studies set out from a psycholinguistic perspective, they vary considerably in their implementation of psycholinguistic thinking. After presenting the cases, we revisit the purpose and content of psycholinguistically based therapy in general, signposting the dangers as well as the positive directions to which this approach can lead. In the final section, Chapter 5.1, by Maria Black, pulls out some of the common themes which span therapy with both children and adults, and Chapter 5.2, by Jane Marshall, sums up the current potential and limits of psycholinguistic applications in language therapy.

Part 1
Phonological processing

Chapter 1.1
Introduction

SHULA CHIAT

The initial hunch about a child or adult may be that their difficulties lie in phonological processing. The hunch may be based on errors in their speech output. They may produce words which miss the mark phonologically, as in the following examples.

Luke, aged 4:

> [mʌ tæ ju bɔɪ mɪ wʌ pi mʌ]
> Target = 'Mum, can you buy me one please mum' (case reported in Chiat 1994)

DJ

> ['emnənt ... 'semənt ... 'tenənt ... 'tenəmən ... 'tɜneɪt]
> Target = 'tenant' (case reported in Butterworth 1992).

Alternatively, their responses to speech input may give rise to the hunch. They may be observed to confuse similar-sounding words, as when William (see Chapter 1.2) took 'dozen' to be 'dustbin' and 'joy' to be 'join'. More extremely, they may show 'word-deafness', as in the case of JS (Caramazza *et al.* 1983) who was almost incapable of understanding spoken words although he performed well with written words.

The most immediate clue to a problem with phonology, then, is the presence of phonological errors in input or output, with segments or syllables within words being omitted, replaced, or transposed. Further grounds for homing in on phonology are:

- The exclusion of difficulties in peripheral sensory and motor processing as the source of the errors: auditory acuity is adequate to perceive speech distinctions, and the structure and function of the vocal organs are adequate to produce speech distinctions.

11

- The exclusion of difficulties with other aspects of words, such as word semantics, as the source of the errors: other aspects of lexical processing may be no problem at all, so that target words, once recognised, are fully appropriate from a semantic and syntactic point of view; alternatively, errors may occur in other aspects of words, suggesting other processing difficulties, but these are ruled out as the source of the phonological errors.

This approach to problems in phonological processing already draws on psycholinguistic thinking in its reference to stages of processing which are or are not involved. Informally, we have distinguished three stages of input and output processing, only one of which is at stake (see Table 1.1.1). This three-way breakdown of word processing is very basic. It enables us to identify a broad range of phonological impairments, but it cannot account for differences between them. This is because the label 'phonology' spans the recognition and planning of complex representations, and impairments may occur at different points in these. The processes and representations involved are by no means simple or obvious, and attempts to characterise them have resulted in numerous models of single word processing. In many cases, these models vary in the terminology they use for different components of processing, rather than in the structures they propose. In some cases, however, the differences are significant.

Table 1.1.1 Stages of input and output processing

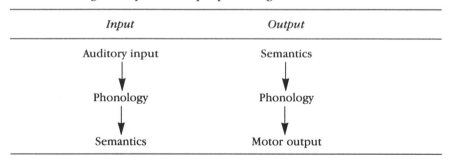

Input	*Output*
Auditory input	Semantics
↓	↓
Phonology	Phonology
↓	↓
Semantics	Motor output

A typical example is the model presented in 1.1.1 (Patterson and Shewell 1987). This model provides a breakdown of spoken word processing, as well as processing of written words. The processing subsumed above under 'phonology' is here divided into lexical and non-lexical components. Spoken input undergoes acoustic analysis which feeds into the **auditory input lexicon** in which word phonologies are stored. In spoken output, word phonology is accessed from the **phonological output lexicon**, and sent to a **response buffer**. The non-lexical pathway provides a direct route between acoustic analysis in input and the response buffer in output, bypassing lexical processing.

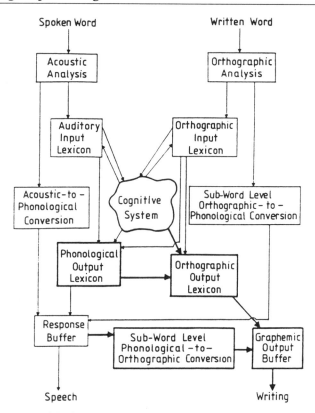

Figure 1.1.1 Model of word and non-word processing (Patterson and Shewell 1987).

This allows us to discriminate and repeat non-words, which have not been stored. The lexical route, on the other hand, allows us to recognise, understand, and name real words which have been stored. It might also be used to discriminate and repeat real words. On the other hand, since discrimination and repetition do not require reference to stored forms, they could be carried out by the non-lexical route. As well as accounting for these possibilities in normal processing, the inclusion of lexical and non-lexical routes accounts for dissociations between the processing of words and non-words which may be observed in cases of impairment. For example, we may find that someone is able to discriminate and repeat real words, but not non-words. The implication is that they are relying on the lexical route to distinguish words and to repeat them, and that the non-lexical route was not available to them. Conversely, we may find that someone is able to discriminate and repeat real words and non-words, implying that the peripheral acoustic and articulatory processing required by the non-lexical route are intact. This person, on the other hand, has difficulties recognising, understanding and naming real words. The implication here is that the lexical route is in some way impaired. This would lead us to look at representations in the input or output phonological lexicons or in the cognitive system.

The architecture of single word processing proposed by others, such as Forster (1976) or Levelt (1992), is similar in most respects. One respect in which they may differ significantly is in the relationship they posit between phonological representations in input and output. Not all models assume separate input and output lexicons. Butterworth (1980), for example, proposes a single phonological lexicon. Levelt's (1992) model of lexical access in speech production draws on a lexicon containing word forms (**lexemes**) and word meanings (**lemmas**). According to both models, the same phonological representation is accessed whether the word is received or produced.

Another difference between models is that some go further than others. Models of speech production, for example, may break down the phonological representation of the word into syllabic, prosodic and segmental aspects (Butterworth 1992).

Similar issues arise in developmental models of speech processing. In some cases, the addressing of these issues in the developmental context may serve to clarify and refine acquired models. Speech processing is one aspect of children's language processing which has received considerable psycholinguistic attention and modelling (e.g. Menn 1983, Spencer 1988, Hewlett 1990, Menn and Matthei 1992, Stackhouse and Wells forthcoming). Developmental models, like adult models, separate out peripheral sensorimotor processing, processing of non-lexical aspects of phonology, and processing of lexical phonology. Again, they allow for a lexical route to ouput, via the stored semantic or phonological representation of a word, and a non-lexical route to output which bypasses the lexical representation.

Like adult models, developmental models vary on the issue of a single lexicon versus separate lexicons for input and output. Most make a distinction between input and output representations. In some cases, this takes the form of separate input and output lexicons (e.g. Hewlett 1990). In others, separate components are distinguished by the representations they contain, e.g. Stackhouse and Wells (forthcoming) refer to a **phonological representation** which is accessed in input, and a **motor programme** which is retrieved in output. Menn and Matthei (1992) combine these with an **input lexicon** identified as a recognition store, and an **output lexicon** identified as a production store. This not only implies that different representations are employed in input and output, but that the output representation contains information specific to articulation. Similarly, Hewlett distinguishes between phonological representations which are perceptually based (input lexicon) and phonological representations which are articulatorily based (output lexicon). The claim is that once the child has worked out a motor programme for a word, this is stored and can be accessed directly. If children do store motor programmes for words in this way, this should be evident in adult processing and reflected in adult models. This is compatible with adult models which incorporate a separate output lexicon, and a direct route from semantic representations to output representations, and implies that those output representations include articulatory information. It is also consistent with dissociations found in adult processing.

Finally, like adult models, developmental models vary when it comes to further breakdown of each stage. For example, Hewlett (1990), like Butterworth (1992), breaks down his motor programme stage into syllabic and segmental aspects.

The similarity between developmental and adult models is striking, perhaps surprisingly so. One might expect the 'developmental dimension' (see the General introduction) to lead to differences in processing models. The similarity may arise from the fact that, by and large, developmental models characterise the system the child is establishing, rather than the process of establishing it. The models themselves say little about the way that one component may affect or be affected by another in the course of development. They say even less about how features within one component, e.g. semantics, may affect features in another component, e.g. phonology. Such issues are taken up in discussion which accompanies the models. We have already seen this in the positing of the output lexicon as the product of connections between semantic representations and motor programmes.

Once we start using these speech processing models, whether child- or adult-related, to explore development or breakdown of speech processing, questions about the internal structure of each component and the interrelations between components arise. In this way, research on disordered phonology contributes to the refinement - and perhaps ultimately re-thinking – of the models.

In the case of development, research has focused on difficulties in output (see Chiat 1994 for an overview). Investigations into the speech of children who mispronounce words have, for example, identified difficulties in the child's output representations of words (Bryan and Howard 1992) and difficulties in their motor programming of words (Chiat 1983, Brett et al. 1987). Detailed analysis of those difficulties has led to further insights into the organisation of lexical representations and their articulation in children.

Interestingly, even though difficulties have in the main been located in output, therapy programmes for phonologically impaired children have tended to focus on input. Therapies in the Bryan and Howard study (1992), the metaphon approach (Dean and Howell 1986, Dean et al. 1995), and the auditory bombardment approach (Hodson and Paden 1983) draw largely on listening and judgement tasks, which involve input processing. In some cases, these are supplemented by self-judgement tasks, where output is required, but the focus is on the child's input processing of that output. The relationship between the input tasks used and the child's difficulties in output is not on the whole discussed explicitly in these studies. The implied assumption, though, is that active manipulation of intact input will have effects either directly on output, or on self-monitoring and hence on output.

In the case of adults with acquired disorders, psycholinguistic work has focused far more on phonological representations of words (see references and discussion in Part 2) than on speech processing. This difference between the developmental and acquired fields could reflect a bias in the interests of therapists or researchers. It could, on the other hand, reflect differences in the deficits which occur during versus following development. For example, it may be that output phonology is susceptible to certain impairments or effects of impairment while lexical representations are being established, but not once they have been established. It may be that impairments at stages of speech processing which are less dependent on lexical representations are more likely to occur in both children and adults. The impairments which lie behind the traditional diagnosis of developmental and acquired dyspraxia may be a case in point. Such impairments invite further exploration to discover which stages of speech processing are implicated, and whether there are indeed parallels between children and adults.

The two chapters which follow pick up these issues at a different stage in the processing story. The child and two adults presented show difficulties with **input** phonology. Here, we might expect to encounter similarities in the peripheral stages of their input processing, but we would surely expect such difficulties to have different ramifications for the child who is acquiring lexical representations and the adults who have acquired them. Each of the following chapters explores the nature of the individuals' difficulties, the motivation for the therapist's intervention, and the effects of that intervention. We turn now to these therapy case studies.

Chapter 1.2
Christopher Lumpship: developing phonological representations in a child with an auditory processing deficit

MAGGIE VANCE

The case reported in this paper is an unusual one. William has a speech and language difficulty arising from the acquired paediatric neurological condition known as **Landau–Kleffner syndrome**. This condition is characterised by the loss of language skills in a child with previous normal development, accompanied by some epileptic manifestations, observable on an electroencephalogram (EEG) but not always resulting in overt seizures. Willliam has a marked auditory processing difficulty that has resulted in multiple errors in speech production. These will be discussed in more detail, and the underlying deficits in speech processing skills identified, as a prelude to describing the therapy programme devised for him.

There are several hypotheses about the nature of the auditory processing deficits found in patients with Landau–Kleffner syndrome. Stephanatos (1991) refers to a difficulty in 'processing specific features of speech sounds critical for language comprehension', whereas Rapin *et al.* (1977) liken the condition to an acquired word deafness when there is a 'deficit for decoding the phonology of acoustic language'. A detailed neuropsychological and neurolinguistic study of an 11 year old boy, whose language deteriorated at age 3, is reported by Denes *et al.* (1986). In this study two hypotheses are considered: whether the child's impairment is the result of

- an inability to process speech at the level of phonetic analysis, although phonological skills are intact, or
- difficulty with phonological analysis of speech.

Findings support evidence of a deficit at a phonetic level of auditory analysis, with difficulty in discriminating and identifying single

17

phonemes. However, at a phonological level, there was also difficulty in discriminating words in a same/different auditory discrimination task, and in judging whether spoken stimuli were words or non-words, in a lexical decision task. The child showed only partial success at an auditory discrimination task when pictures were presented, suggesting he was reliant on semantic mediation and top-down processing to support discrimination. However, it is not clear whether lower-level difficulties in auditory processing were also responsible for impaired performance at a phonological level, or whether a more central phonological impairment was present. Comparison of such cases with children with a hearing loss, where the auditory deficit is clearly peripheral in nature would help to resolve this issue. Bishop (1982) showed that children with Landau–Kleffner syndrome made the same kind of consistent errors on comprehension tasks as deaf children, which indicates that their language difficulties might be the result of a more peripheral auditory processing deficit.

There are few reports of therapy carried out with children with this difficulty. The use of the visual channel to present linguistic information in a written or signed format has been advocated (Worster-Drought 1971, Huskisson 1973, Rapin et al. 1977, Ferry and Cooper 1978, Suzuki and Notoya 1980, De Wijngaert and Gommers 1993). Gerard et al. (1991) report details of therapy carried out with a 13 year old child (8 years after the deterioration of language skills). One aim of therapy was to use lip-reading skills and visual forms of known words for decoding to 'fixate lexical representations the child could use without the necessary passage through auditory analysis' and the development of associations between spoken word and written word. Over a 9 month period of attendance in special education provision with twice daily speech therapy, gains were made in the child's naming and word repetition skills and in intelligibility but there was no improvement in verbal comprehension. The progress reported is explained in terms of the Ellis and Young (1988) speech processing model as short-circuiting channels through auditory analysis, with recreation of links from the visual input lexicon to the semantic system and speech output lexicon. Gerard et al. (1991) summarise their approach to therapy in such cases as 'building communication from oral residues' rather than from dysfunction. This is in contrast to the approach of Dugas (1972), described by Gerard et al. (1991), in which there is direct intervention on the 'sensory' deficit, with work on auditory and phonetic discrimination and the construction of an oral input lexicon. This dichotomy illustrates a recurring theme in the discussion and planning of speech and language therapy: whether the therapy programme should build on a child's existing strengths or target the weaknesses within his speech and language system. The therapy programme planned for William and described in this paper utilises the strengths in his speech processing profile but also targets the weaknesses.

Subject information

Developmental history

William had a history of normal development and his verbal language was developing within the normal range. At the age of 3 years 6 months his language skills rapidly deteriorated and this symptom, in association with characteristic spiking patterns on his EEG, led to the diagnosis of Landau–Kleffner syndrome. After treatment with steroid medication, the irregularities observed on EEG recordings had ceased, but language did not recover. At later medical investigations, no abnormality was detected on magnetic resonance scanning, and subsequent EEGs were normal. Following the loss of language skills, William had auditory agnosia. Environmental sounds were meaningless; for example he could not detect the difference between a doorbell and a phone ringing. He did not understand any spoken language and his expressive language was reduced to jargon-like patterns with intonation contours. It is possible that this deterioration of William's own speech was the result of break-down in the auditory feedback mechanisms that support self-monitoring of speech output.

Family and social information

William is an only child, with a very supportive family unit. Both parents are in work. William has good friends in his neighbourhood, so spends much of his leisure time with children who are developing normally. He has similar interests to his peers: computers, roller-blades and discos.

Former therapy

Early therapy involved the use of Makaton signing to promote communication as well as language skills and conceptual development. At the age of 5 years, William attended a primary school for children with severe speech and language disorders. The Paget–Gorman Sign System was used in therapy and social situations, in the classroom and at home. The use of visually presented timetables allowed everyday activities to provide material for the early teaching of signed and written language. An auditory training programme led to the development of some speech recognition skills and limited verbal comprehension and expression. The use of cued articulation (see page 33) provided visual support for the teaching of phonological distinctions between words. Further details of these educational and therapy programmes and subsequent progress have previously been reported by Vance (1991).

When William was 8 years old he transferred to a unit for hearing-impaired children that was attached to a mainstream school. Signing support was available to all children along with specialised teaching, and some sessions of integration into mainstream classes. Speech and language therapy involvement was confined to an assessment and monitoring role. Over the period of a year, William's verbal language showed considerable improvement and his dependency on signing diminished, so that he was no longer reliant on it for communication or for language learning. He transferred again to a school for deaf children that did not use signing within the school, but followed a programme within the oral tradition of deaf education. Again there was no direct speech and language therapy involvement for the first 18 months. During the course of this educational placement the therapy programme described in this paper was implemented.

Speech and language skills

At the commencement of this period of therapy William was 10 years old. He was a keen communicator with good social skills, using spoken language, although not always intelligible. Expressive language was characterised by the use of simple sentences with syntactic errors and omissions, vocabulary was also reduced. However, William could use long strings of such utterances to tell quite lengthy, detailed stories and to give relevant information.

T: You've got some more rabbits.
W: Yeh. You know Billy and James? You know.
T: You had two rabbits last time I came.
W: But it's gone.
T: Where ?
W: James leave it because ... if I put ... long time ago when small like [lʌdən] Billy and James like together in a ... in a hutch. And play it and play it, but ...when it get big like a man yeh? And do you know you fight together... you get killed ... like ... I din know you know James [liv] it. I din know. My dad take James in a work and give a lady [æwɛlə] bring it back.
T: So how many rabbits have you got?
W: I got one rabbit Billy, and I go ... that's Mum rabbit that's Mum.
T: That's Mum's rabbit?
W: Yeh. A white one got brown. His name ... Patch and it's got all brown it's got white.
T: So all his body is brown?
W: Got everywhere brown and it's got white somewhere, somewhere, I not sure somewhere and that's it.

William frequently misunderstood verbal language and had difficulty processing longer utterances that were spoken to him. He often misperceived words heard and this had implications for comprehension. Examples arose during a psychological assessment that included William asking 'you mean dustbin?' when the word 'dozen' was used, 'joy' being mistaken as 'join' and the word 'leave' defined by William as 'on a tree full of leaves'.

William produced many words inaccurately. Some errors showed consistency in the type of substitutions and omissions being made across words. These included:

- Substitution of /t/ and /d/ for /k/ and /g/
  e.g. give→[dɪv], case→[teɪs], garden→[dɑdn̩], duck→[dʌt], bag→[bæd], together→[tədɛvə], sugar→[ʃʊdə], fox→[fɒt]

- Reduction of affricates
  e.g. chair→[sɛə], chase([teɪs]

- Omission of final consonants
  e.g. tent→[tɛn], pipe →[pɔɪʔ], dark→[dɑʔ], red→[rɛʔ], mrs→[mɪsɪ]

- Reduction in clusters
  e.g. slide→[saɪd], blue→[bu], clock→[kɒʔ], school→[sul], loads→[ləʊz]

- Omission of syllables
  e.g. Victoria→[tɪtɔrə], moustache→[ʃtæʃ], zebra→[zɛg]

- Errors in sequencing phonemes within words
  e.g. upset→[ʌpstɛʔ], juggle→[dɛldl]

However, other errors were more idiosyncratic and word-specific. For example:

sea-saw→[swɪŋsɒk], light-house→[laɪtɪŋ]
Christopher Columbus→[fɪsəfə lʌmpʃɪp]

William has some distortion and substitution of vowels and diph-thongs in his own speech production. William's parents have a Scottish accent in which many vowels are differently realised from those commonly used in south-east England where the family lived and William attended school. This had made analysis of William's vowel system complex. He was using some vowels as appropriate to a southern English accent, some vowels were realised as would have been expected within a Scottish accent and some vowel realisations fitted neither accent pattern. However the vowel system was judged to be less impaired than William's use of consonants and was not systematically addressed in therapy at this time.

Standardised assessment results

Psychological assessment (William aged 10 years 8 months)

Wechsler Intelligence Scale for Children III (UK) (Wechsler 1992)

Verbal scaled score	62
Performance scaled score	95

Wechsler Objective Reading Dimensions (Rust *et al*. 1993)

Basic Reading scaled score	69	age equivalent	6;09
Spelling scaled score	67	age equivalent	6;09
Reading Comprehension scaled score	62	age equivalent	6;06

Speech and Language Assessment (William aged 10)

British Picture Vocabulary Scales (Dunn *et al*. 1982)
The British Picture Vocabulary Scales is a standardised assessment of receptive vocabulary. The child selects which of four pictures corresponds with the spoken word presented to him.

Standard score	47	age equivalent	4;06

Test for Reception of Grammar (Bishop 1982)
The Test for the Reception of Grammar is a standardised test of a child's comprehension of sentence forms. The child is presented with four pictures and has to identify the one that illustrates the sentence that is spoken.

Standard score	66	age equivalent	5;04

Clinical Evaluation of Language Fundamentals (Semel *et al*. 1980)
The Clinical Evaluation of Language Fundamentals has a number of sub-tests. The Word Structure sub-test examines the child's ability to supply a word with an appropriate morphological suffix in a sentence cloze procedure. The Oral Directions sub-test presents the child with a series of commands requiring the child to point to one or more of a series of shapes. Understanding a paragraph is a sub-test in which a short story is read out to the child, who is then asked some questions about the story.

Word Structure sub-test standard score	3
Oral Directions sub-test standard score	3
Understanding a Paragraph sub-test standard score	4

(An average standard score would be 10. William's scores on these sub-tests are therefore significantly below normal limits for his age.) Speech errors may have affected scoring of some responses in the Word Structure sub-test. For example: For a correct response of 'Ann's', William's response was [ænd], and it was unclear if the /d/ represented /z/ or not. For a correct response 'noisy', William's response was [nɔtɪ], and it was unclear if William meant 'naughty' or 'noisy'.

Reading and spelling

William's performance on the Wechsler Objective Reading Dimensions suggested his reading and spelling skills were at about a 6 year 6 month level. He was heavily reliant on visual strategies for reading and spelling, with some use of phonic strategies just emerging. For example, when reading aloud he would either recognise a word or guess at it using context and the initial letter, but with no correspondence to the rest of the written word. In the spelling of CVC nonsense words, William used the correct initial consonant, but incorrect final consonants.

Psycholinguistic assessment

As the basis for the planning and implementation of a therapy programme some details of assessment findings are considered. It is only through thorough investigation of speech processing skills that a clear rationale for the therapy programme can be obtained. A psycholinguistic approach to assessment was taken as this would allow strengths and weaknesses within the speech processing system to be identified and these would influence the choice of tasks and techniques involved in the therapy programme.

William's speech and lexical difficulties were analysed in terms of a psycholinguistic assessment framework (Stackhouse and Wells 1993, forthcoming), which distinguishes between different levels of processing of speech input and speech output and the integrity of phonological representations (see Figure 1.2.1). The framework consists of a series of questions that can be posed to enable the level, or levels, of deficits in speech processing that underlie speech difficulties to be identified (see Figure 1.2.2). Although it seems obvious from the history and the observation of frequent misperception that William's speech and language difficulties could be explained by his auditory processing deficit, profiling his speech processing skills allows these deficits to be more precisely defined. A more detailed description and discussion of some of the tasks used to profile speech processing skills can be found in Vance (1996). The following questions from the psycholinguistic assessment framework were addressed.

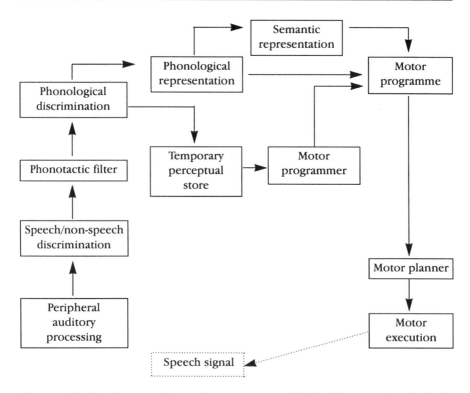

Figure 1.2.1 Developmental speech processing model (Stackhouse and Wells forthcoming).

Speech input processing

Does the child have adequate pre-linguistic auditory perception?

Regular audiological testing was carried out at school and indicated that William did not have any significant hearing loss. He was now able to identify environmental sounds that were similar, for example cars, buses and aeroplanes. It is possible that William would have had some difficulty in discriminating finer differences in non-verbal sounds, in discriminating between tones of different pitches for example, but such testing was not carried out.

Can the child discriminate speech sounds without reference to his/her own phonological representations?

William found non-word auditory discrimination tasks difficult, and made frequent errors. In one task, non-word stimuli were presented using two soft toys. The task used an ABX design, with the format '(He says) /brɪʃ/, (He says) /brɪs/, (Which one said) /brɪs/?'. The carrier phrases were used to introduce the task but were faded out before the test items. On this task William made only a few errors with one-syllable

PSYCHOLINGUISTIC ASSESSMENT OF CHILDREN WITH SPEECH
AND LITERACY DIFFICULTIES

Joy Stackhouse and Bill Wells

PSYCHOLINGUISTIC PROFILE SUMMARY SHEET

Name: William   DOB: Date: CA: 10 years

INPUT

F. Is the child aware of the internal structure of phonological representations?
No

E. Are the child's phonological representations accurate?
No

D. Can the child detect similarities and differences between real words?
No

C. Does the child have language-specific representations of word structures?
–

B. Can the child discriminate speech sounds without reference to his/her own phonological representations?
No

A. Does the child have adequate pre-linguistic auditory perception?
Yes

OUTPUT

G. Can the child produce his/her phonological representations accurately?
Yes

H. Can the child manipulate phonological units?
No

I. Can the child articulate real words accurately?
Yes

J. Can the child articulate connected utterances fluently?
Yes

K. Can the child articulate speech without reference to his/her phonological representations?
No (but see discussion re: effects of input processing on performance)

I. Does the child have adequate non-linguistic sound production?
Yes

GENERAL COMMENTS

Figure 1.2.2 Psycholinguistic assessment framework (based on Stackhouse and Wells 1997, forthcoming) with William's performance indicated.

non-words (scored 17/20), but he performed at a chance level when non-words of two or more syllables were used (scored 11/20). A same/different task consisted of a selection from the stimuli devised by Bridgeman and Snowling (1988). Most of William's errors involved non-word pairs where there was a sequence change in the final cluster, for example *kest/kets* (scored 14/18), rather than a contrast between two single consonant codas, for example *kes/ket* (scored 17/18).

Can the child detect similarities and differences between real words?

William made a similar number of errors in a same/different auditory discrimination task when words rather than non-words were used. A similar set of stimuli was selected from the Bridgeman and Snowling (1988) list, and, as with the non-word list, revealed more difficulty with sequence changes, e.g. *rates/raced* (scored 13/18), than with single consonant changes, e.g. *rate/race* (scored 17/18). William needed frequent repetitions, and was observed to be lip-reading while participating in another same/different task using a set of minimal pairs with plosive contrasts, such as *bike/bite* and *lock/log*.

Are the child's phonological representations accurate?

William also made errors when he had to compare correct and incorrect pronunciations of the names of pictures. In an auditory-visual lexical decision task (after Locke 1980), he was shown a picture and asked to judge whether the name for the picture was said correctly or not, for example, 'Is this right, "brush"?' or 'Is this right, /brʌs/?' William scored 63/96. The Auditory Discrimination and Attention Test (Morgan-Barry 1988) is a picture minimal pair task in which the child is shown two pictures depicting a minimal pair, e.g. *pear/bear*, and asked to point to the one spoken by the tester. William's error score of 35 places him well below normal limits (for 5 year old children the mean error score is 8). Auditory input tasks such as these, which involve the use of pictures, required William to compare the spoken form of the word with his own phonological representation(s) of the picture or pictures, in order to judge what was heard. His reduced performance here suggested that representations were not always accurate. However, the difficulty he was having with lower levels of input processing would also affect performance on such tasks.

Although not all potential contrasts were sampled in these two tasks, many of the errors made reflected those in William's own speech, such as confusion with presentations of words containing /k/ and /t/, affricates and blends. There were a few errors when metathetic changes had been made to words and an error on the one instance when the final consonant was omitted.

Is the child aware of the internal structure of phonological represen-tations?

William was able to identify correctly the initial or final consonants of some words represented by pictures, for example, p̲an, m̲ilk, hook̲, bed̲ (scored 6/10). However, he sometimes seemed to rely on visual, ortho-graphic knowledge to do this, so that his response for the picture of 'chicken' was that it began with /k/, and initial phonemes were some-times identified by their letter names, rather than phoneme. For example, asked what sound *frog* began with, William responded /ɛf/. William was at a chance level in judging whether two words rhymed or not, when presented with pictures of the word.

Speech output processing

Can the child produce his/her phonological representations accurately?

In naming pictures and in spontaneous speech, William was consistent in his pronunciation of words. The errors that William made in his spon-taneous speech matched the errors that he made in auditory discrimi-nation tasks. This suggests his speech errors may reflect inaccurate phonological representations, and that these inaccuracies stem from auditory processing difficulties. For example, William tended to use /t/ instead of /k/ in spoken words and confused this contrast in auditory discrimination tasks such as identifying whether *key* or *tea* was spoken in a picture presentation minimal pair task.

Can the child manipulate phonological units?

William found it difficult to generate rhyming strings and tended to give semantically related responses, for example when asked to find a rhyme for 'spoon' he responded 'sugar'. He sometimes relied on visual, ortho-graphic knowledge to help him, so that when asked to produce a rhyme for 'boy' William traced the word out on the table with his finger, and responded 'yo-yo – no that the wrong way round'. He was only able to generate a very limited number of words that began or ended with a particular phoneme. He used a strategy of looking around the room for ideas, and so relying on semantic mediation to access words before deciding whether they began with the target phoneme or not.

Can the child articulate real words accurately?

William was often more accurate in his production of words in a repeti-tion task than in a naming task, for example *crab* was named as [præt] but imitated as [kræb], *fish* named as [ʃɪʃ] but imitated as [fɪʃ]. Scores on speech production tasks reflected this with 16/20 completely accurate productions on repetition and 13/20 on naming for single-syllable words. So when William did not have to rely on his own (inaccurate) phonological representations to say words he was more successful. It would seem that William was able to make some distinctions auditorily that were not specified in his representations. This also demonstrated that he had the necessary output skills to articulate these words correctly, since he could produce the word correctly on repetition. Thus, his speech production errors were occurring at the level of phonological representations, rather than at a more peripheral level of output processing.

Can the child articulate speech without reference to his/her phonological representations?

Repetition of non-words was often very inaccurate, and deteriorated with increased length of the non-words (scoring 9/20 accurate productions for one-syllable non-words and 2/20 for non-words of 3–4 syllables). In view of William's improved performance on repetition of words, as compared to naming, this illustrates that he was heavily reliant on the lexical support provided by existing semantic and phonological representations. Additional auditory information could supplement his existing phonological knowledge but in the absence of this knowledge he experienced considerable difficulty in perceiving and identifying the phonemes in the speech that he heard, so that he was often unable to gain enough information about the phonological content of the sound string to produce a recognisable repetition. William tended to lexicalise responses, for example /plǝut/ was repeated as 'float'. This provides further evidence for lack of specification in the phonological representations leading him to 'recognise' non-words as words, even though task instructions indicated that he would hear made-up words. Although poor motor programming skills might explain poor non-word repetition, in William's case errors were arising from input processing deficits.

Does the child have adequate non-linguistic sound production?

William did not show any evidence of difficulty with oromotor movements.

Conclusions from psycholinguistic investigations

In summary, William's speech processing profile indicated that he continued to have difficulty with auditory discrimination of both known words and non-words. This had resulted in the laying down of inaccurate phonological representations. The source of William's

speech errors lay in the inaccuracy of his phonological representations (inaccuracies arising as a consequence of his auditory processing difficulties) and the inaccurate motor programmes for words that
had been derived from these faulty phonological representations.
Subsequent stages of output processing would seem to be intact. He
was also relying on visual information using contextual clues, and top-
down processing using existing linguistic knowledge, to assist in
decoding the speech signal and thus support weak input processing
skills. William had developed some phonological awareness skills,
particularly in the identification of the onset of some words, but was
having difficulty with other aspects of phonological awareness such as
rhyme.

The developmental speech processing model (Stackhouse and Wells,
forthcoming) can be used to illustrate the deficits in William's speech
processing skills (Figure 1.2.1). It would seem that William had some
difficulty at the level of phonological discrimination and phonological
representations, together with their motor programmes, but that motor
programmer, motor planning and motor execution skills were relatively
intact. The assessments carried out were not fine enough to rule out an
auditory processing deficit at a more peripheral level than phonological
discrimination. However, William was successful in discriminating
between some phoneme contrasts and minimal pairs, suggesting that if
a deficit at a peripheral level was present, its effect on the perception of
speech sounds was selective and not universal. The presence of relatively adequate speech recognition suggests that William was capable of
speech/non-speech discrimination. Investigations of processing of non-
verbal sound in other groups of children with speech processing
deficits, e.g. developmental language disorder (Tallal and Piercy 1973)
and dyslexia (Masterson *et al*. 1995), suggest that deficits at this peripheral level of input processing are present. It is quite possible that
William had difficulty in perceiving fine differences in all sound, not just
in speech. Further investigations to cover this possibility are currently
being planned.

Implications for semantic and phonological representations

As a consequence of such marked auditory processing difficulties,
William had come to rely on top-down processing, and the use of
contextual and semantic knowledge, in order to perceive and recognise speech signals. He also made use of visually presented information, such as orthography. However, these particular coping strategies
have compounded his difficulty in creating accurate phonological
representations in various ways. For instance, the use of orthographic

cues has resulted in some of the phonological information about a word being derived from its spelling rather than from its spoken form, so that the car name *Porche* was pronounced as [pɔtʃ] rather than the more usual /pɔʃ/, because of the 'ch' present in the spelling of the word.

The use of semantic cues has also resulted in the creation of inaccurate phonological representations. One such example is William's word 'Christopher Lumpship', [ˈfɪsəfə ˈlʌmpʃɪp], for 'Christopher Columbus' where some of the phonology of the word, i.e. /lʌmp/, is combined with semantic information associated with the character, i.e. that he travelled in a ship. Another example is [ˈlæbədɒg] for 'Labrador', where again semantic information, that this is the name of a breed of dog, supplements the recognised sounds that have been stored from hearing the word.

The auditory processing difficulties have also affected semantic representation. Sometimes when a known word was heard it was not recognised as a word with an existing lexical entry. This prevented the semantic representations from being updated by the additional semantic information gained from hearing words used in different contexts. Additionally, there were times when a new word was perceived as being the same as an existing known word. The semantic information relating to the new word became incorporated into the semantic representation of the existing lexical item. An example of this arose when William referred to Captain Hook as 'a pirate who went around planting the English flag'. William had seen a recent film about the pirate Captain Hook from the Peter Pan story, and then heard in school about the exploits of Captain Cook. It is supposed that, recognising the new name of 'Captain Cook' as 'Captain Hook' the new semantic information given became amalgamated with the existing representation to create the character that William described. This explanation for some errors in word usage might also account for William's naming of a polar bear as [kɒlə bɛə]. The familiar label *koala bear* may have been accessed in the semantic context of a *polar bear*, so that the two semantic representations become assimilated with a single phonological representation.

Implications for morphology

William had some concept of appropriate morphology, of plural and past tense, for instance, as evidenced by his use of appropriate sign and in his written work. However, the phonological content of morphological suffixes was not often signalled in his speech output. The deletion of final consonants and weak syllables that characterises some of William's speech output would lead to omission of morphological endings. It has already been reported that William had markedly more difficulty in discriminating the differences in sequence changes of final clusters than differences between single final consonants. This discriminatory difficulty would also mitigate against the development of clear representations of the phonological changes required to signal morphological information, as in many instances, these are marked by final clusters.

Therapy hypotheses

Therapy targeted at developing more accurate phonological representations should lead to a reduction in speech output errors. This would require the visual presentation of phonological information to support the continuing auditory discrimination deficits. More accurate phonological representations should, in turn, lead to increased awareness of differences between words and less misperception of speech signals heard, aiding recognition and comprehension.

Aims for therapy

Four main aims were considered in devising a therapy programme for William:

1. To revise his inaccurate phonological representations and the accompanying motor programmes as this should result in more intelligible speech and fewer speech errors.
2. To increase William's awareness and discrimination of the phoneme contrasts and clusters that he did not seem to be perceiving consistently, so that the phonology for new lexical items would be more accurately perceived and stored, and words heard would be more readily recognised.
3. To promote phonological awareness skills, which would also allow more accurate analysis of the phonology of existing and new words, and support the development of phonological strategies for reading and spelling development.
4. To provide phonological details of morphological suffixes, to allow these to be incorporated into spontaneous speech.

Therapy regime

William was seen by the speech and language therapist for one session each week over a 2 year period. Each session lasted approximately 45 minutes. Details of activities that reinforced areas worked on in each session were left for William to work through on his own or with one of his parents.

Therapy programme

General considerations

It was clear from William's speech processing profile that phonological information about words should be presented in a visual format to support his poor auditory discrimination skills. Visual support would also be needed for auditory discrimination tasks, until discrimination skills had developed further.

Speech output processing skills were unimpaired and could be used for rehearsal of the correct articulation of phonemes and words from visual cues. This would allow William to become aware of phoneme contrasts that he was having difficulty discriminating, for example /k/ and /t/. It would also provide bottom-up feedback through the speech output processing chain to update motor programmes. It is hypothesised that revision of motor programmes could also have a knock-back effect on phonological representations, thus working from production to aid discrimination (see Figure 1.2.3).

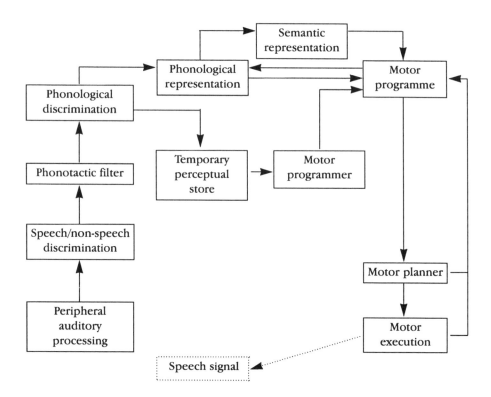

Figure 1.2.3 Speech processing model (Stackhouse and Wells forthcoming), with arrows to indicate feedback from speech output to motor programme and phonological representations.

Words and phoneme contrasts to be included in therapy activities were collected from analysis of errors that occurred in William's speech, many of which were somewhat idiosyncratic. For all errors that were targeted, William had opportunities to take turns as both speaker and listener in activities, so that speech production and discrimination skills were being developed in parallel.

Most of the materials and word-lists used were generated by William himself or taken from his own speech. This allowed therapy activities to utilise words that William himself used and that were meaningful and relevant to him. This was considered to be important to keep motivation high and therapy relevant. William is a keen and talented young artist. Many of the pictorial illustrations used in therapy activities were prepared by himself.

Cued articulation

Visual support for speech production and auditory discrimination was achieved by using the **cued articulation** technique (Passy 1990) and orthographic representations of words. Cued articulation allows each individual phoneme of English to be represented by a hand posture that denotes information about some of the features of the phoneme, e.g. place and manner of articulation and voicing (Figure 1.2.4). The system also incorporates the use of differently coloured lines to underline the letters of a written word and indicate the phoneme that each corresponds to in the spoken form of the word. So, for example, the 'k' in *king* and the 'c' in *cat* would both be underlined in the colour brown to represent the phoneme /k/, the 'c' in *circle* and the 's' in *sun* would both be underlined in pale green to represent the phoneme /s/, while the 's' in *sugar* and the 'sh' in *shop* would both be underlined in red representing /ʃ/. This dual visual representation of the phonemes within a word illustrated that although there are observable phoneme/ grapheme correspondences in English orthography, the sequence of sounds of a word is not always exactly the same as the sequence of letters used to write it. This was felt to be an important distinction to make in helping William to analyse the phonology of words, without relying solely on their orthography to do so.

The cued articulation scheme was re-introduced to William in its entirety, as it had not been used with him for the previous 2 years. Each individual hand posture was demonstrated, with the photograph of the posture retained as a cue. A list of words containing the phoneme in different positions was generated in discussion and written down, with the appropriate letters underlined in the appropriate colours. As William found it difficult to think of words that began or ended with a particular sound, he was given semantic clues to help him guess some examples. This allowed him to be involved in creating the materials used in this therapy activity. Contrasting orthographic representations were included where possible, for example 'f/ff/ph/gh' (see Figure 1.2.4). All the consonants were introduced in this way and their production practised.

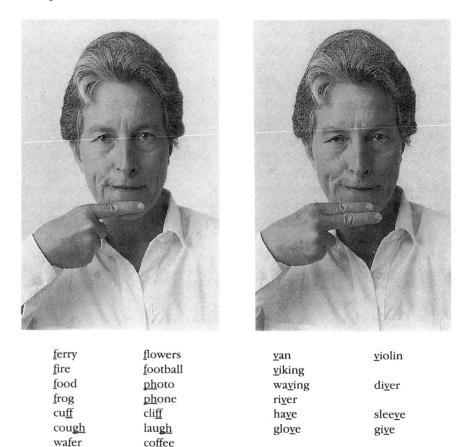

ferry	flowers	van	violin
fire	football	viking	
food	photo	waving	diver
frog	phone	river	
cuff	cliff	have	sleeve
cough	laugh	glove	give
wafer	coffee		
office			

Figure 1.2.4 Examples of hand postures used in cued articulation (Passy 1990), with set of words used to illustrate the phonemes in different contexts in words, and with differerent spellings used. (In the original the letters representing /f/ and /v/ are underlined in pink.) (From Passy, J. Cued Articulation (1990) Reproduced by permission of The Australian Council for Educational Research Ltd.)

Refining phonological representations and auditory discrimination

Word-specific errors

With this background knowledge of cued articulation hand postures and practice in the production of single consonants, word-specific errors were tackled for individual words. Visual feedback was given for the correct sequence of phonemes for the word through the written form of both the correct and incorrect version of the word, with the relevant letters underlined, the use of cued articulation hand postures to give visual cues and feedback to correct articulation. For example, *rabbit* was consistently produced as [rædɪt]. Two versions of the word *rabbit* and *raddit* were written out with the 'bb' and 'dd' underlined in colour as appropriate for /b/ and /d/. The differences between the two versions of the word were discussed and ticks and crosses showed which was the correct and which the incorrect version (see Figure 1.2.5). This was followed by practice in saying the word with the correct pronunciation, feedback being given in the form of cued articulation, lip-reading cues and the orthographic forms.

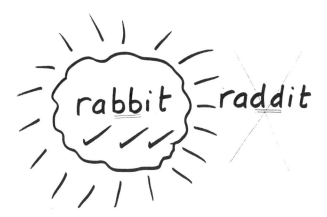

Figure 1.2.5 How orthographic forms of correct and incorrect pronunciations were used to give feedback in therapy. (In the original, letters representing /b/ and /d/ are underlined in orange and pale blue.)

For auditory discrimination practice, William pointed to the version of the word that was spoken to him (mouth covered), for example 'Which one am I saying, "raddit"?', and he then took turns in saying the two forms of the word for the therapist to point to the version heard. This allowed him to reflect on his own articulation of the word and receive immediate feedback on his production. Later auditory discrimination involved William in giving a thumbs-up if he heard the correct version, and a thumbs-down on hearing the incorrect version. For example, 'Is this right or wrong, "raddit"?' Again William had an opportunity to say the word with the therapist giving thumbs-up and thumbs-down feedback according to whether the word was correct or not. When the therapist was sure that William was able to say the word correctly, and was aware of the difference between his usual error and the desired pronunciation, feedback was given in William's spontaneous conversation if the old pattern was used.

Sometimes the incorrect version of an individual word sounded very like William's production of another word. When this occurred, pictures of the two similar sounding words could be used along with the written forms, cued articulation, etc. For example William's pronunciation of *wizard* sounded very like his production of *whistle*. The same sequence of practising saying the words concerned and discriminating between them was carried out.

Across-word errors

Other errors were more consistent across words. For instance, where /k/ and /g/ should occur in words, they were often realised as /t/ or /d/; final consonants were omitted in many words. For these errors pictures of minimal pair sets containing the relevant phoneme contrasts were drawn by William (Figure 1.2.6). These were used to highlight the difference between the target sound and the sound being substituted, again by using visual support with cued articulation hand postures, orthographic forms, coloured underlines and lip-reading cues.

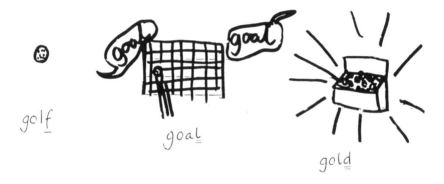

Figure 1.2.6 Illustrations (drawn by William) of minimal pairs with final consonant differences. (In the original, the final letters are underlined in colours appropriate to the phonemes they represent.)

Motor speech skills were utilised in practising articulating each of the minimal pair words to provide bottom-up feedback to motor programmes and to heighten William's awareness of the existence of the two different phonemes and the nature of their differences. For instance, discussion of the differing places of articulation of /k/ and /t/ reinforced lip-reading cues that would be useful in the context of listening. Strings of minimal pairs were practised in sequence, the cue being the written forms with key letters underlined to indicate the phoneme contrasts. For example: key, tea, key, tea, key, tea, key, tea, key, tea, key, tea (ks underlined with a brown line, and ts underlined with a pale blue line). As with articulatory drilling practice, the sequences were made more complex, such as *key, key, tea, key, tea, tea, tea, key, key, tea, tea, key*, to establish the articulatory patterns for the words. To maintain motivation for this repeated activity, score-sheets were used for each practice. These recorded the date and the number of items articulated correctly, so that William was competing against his own previous performance. This was sufficient motivation, and William would often ask for one more chance to 'get them all right'.

Auditory discrimination activities with the minimal pair pictures were carried out with cued articulation and lip-reading cues available when errors were made. First William listened and pointed to the picture he thought he heard named, and then (when he had practised articulation of the words in the pairs sufficiently) William said the words for the therapist to point to the pictures. Later, non-word minimal pairs were presented for same/different auditory discrimination, to develop discrimination skills in the absence of lexical support, for example: /gɒm/, /dɒm/ and /wʌd/, /wʌg/. The same and different non-word pairs were written out on slips of paper, in conventional orthography, which were turned upside-down and mixed up. The therapist would select a slip of paper and read out the non-word pair, mouth covered. William would respond and then be shown the written version to give him feedback as to whether he was right or wrong. Where he had responded incorrectly the non-word pair were repeated with cued articulation and lip-reading cues available.

Pictures were then drawn, and names written with appropriate coloured underlining, of lots of words that contained the target phoneme, for example *cake, carrot, car, king, kettle, caravan*. Use was made of all the visual prompts that had been used previously and William practised saying these words correctly.

Targets tackled in this way included /k, g/ ; /ʃ, tʃ, dʒ /; final consonants; clusters containing /l/; and /st/ and /sk/ clusters. William's auditory discrimination difficulty was very persistent and at times mitigated against success in structured therapy practice. One example of this occurred when working on the minimal pair, *grass/glass*. When these items were introduced William drew a picture of a glass, that is used for drinking. Asked to draw grass, he pointed to the back garden visible through the glass doors to check his interpretation of my request was correct and drew a green square. Subsequently we were practising discrimination of this minimal pair when it became apparent that for William both pictures represented glass, one a drinking glass and the other the glass of the door!

Once William was completely familiar with the production of words and phoneme contrasts targeted in therapy, feedback was given to his spontaneous speech. Frequently what William had said was written down in the same way as he said it, to give immediate visual feedback. William quickly picked up on this strategy and would often self-correct as the mispronounced word was written.

Phonological awareness

Some of the activities carried out as described above were also aiding the development of phonological awareness skills. The orthographic cues and coloured underlining helped to highlight the notion that sounds and letters are not the same thing. William was frequently being asked to reflect on a word under discussion and identify initial and final consonants.

There was some omission of syllables in William's own speech. Improved syllable awareness might be beneficial in aiding analysis of words heard and in updating phonological representations, as well as in developing phonological awareness skills for reading and spelling. Sets of words with the same root-form were written out, marking the syllable boundaries with oblique lines, for example, *fish*, *fish/ing*, *fish/er/man*, and noting the number of syllables alongside. The number of syllables was then clapped out as the words were spoken. A list of animal names, and the names of friends, generated by William, were used for syllable-clapping, moving on to lists of words noted down during conversation at the start of sessions. For example discussion of a school trip yielded *Longleat*, *Youth Hostel*, *dinner*, *hot chocolate*, *Wookey Hole*, *Victoria*, and *horrible packed lunch*, amongst others, for syllable-clapping. Initially words were spoken in time to hand-claps or drumming on the table, with equal stress given to all syllables, William clapping along with the therapist and then directly after. Again the words were written and the number of syllables recorded alongside. Then the words were spoken by the therapist for William to clap out or drum the number of syllables. Previously unpractised words were presented and more natural stress patterns were adopted as awareness of syllables improved. William became quite proficient at this task over a short period of time.

Rhyming skills were also targeted in therapy. Plastic letters were used to construct sequences of rhyming words, using the orthographic cues to show how the rime units of the words were the same. The words were also spoken to show how the words sounded similar. Lists of words that rhymed were constructed showing William how they sounded alike, i.e. rhymed. As well as rhyming pairs and sets that were spelt the same, sets with different spellings were included to draw attention to the 'sound' element of rhyme, and that 'sound' was not the same as spelling. Pictures of words that rhymed were selected from a range of pictures. However, rhyming activities were not very successful with William, possibly because of his own somewhat different vowel system, referred to earlier. William became able to recognise whether two words rhymed or not, but remained unable to generate his own rhyming responses.

Morphology

Work on morphological suffixes consisted of reinforcing their phonological content both in production and in discrimination, that is, the morphophonology. Plural and past-tense endings were targeted.

For plural endings, minimal pair pictures consisting of single and multiple items were used, for example *car/cars*, *horse/horses*, *boot/boots*. Initially CV words and their plural forms were used, and then CVC or CCVC words and their plurals were used, as it was predicted that William would find it more difficult to discriminate the clusters that resulted when a word with a final consonant was pluralised than a plural form resulting in a single consonant. Picture pairs were first presented for auditory discrimination of the singular versus plural items. Again visual cues were used to highlight the sound differences that needed to be attended to. The therapist and William took turns in saying the singular and plural words for each other to select the appropriate picture. The different phonological forms that resulted when forms were pluralised were illustrated, so that William could learn when the plural form would be /s/, when /z/ and when /ɪz/, according to the final phoneme of the singular word. For instance, one worksheet read 'If the word ends with a "s" or "z" sound, we add "es" and say **two** "s" sounds' (*s* and *z* underlined in appropriate colours). A list of words this rule applied to followed, such as *horse/horses*, *face/faces* (final s underlined with pale green). At a later session the written comment 'Also for words that end in "sh" was added, with a list of examples, such as *brush/brushes*, *wish/wishes*.

Similarly with past tenses, lists of verbs were created and sorted according to the phonological form of the past tense ending of /t/, /d/ or /ɪd/. The visual presentations of coloured underlines of the *-ed*, and written forms of the different sounds the past tense forms manifested, reinforced the appropriate phonology. The spoken forms of the past tenses were practised to set up motor programme patterns. The use of the past tense suffix was practised in connected speech by using action pictures and sentences such as: 'Today he's playing with the toy.'; 'Last week he play*ed* (underlined with two pale blue lines to denote /d/) with the toy.' In picture descriptions, starter phrases such as 'Yesterday afternoon' were given to practise use of past tense. A diary format was also used to consolidate this work.

For both plurals and past tenses those words that resulted in an irregular pattern were also practised. William already used some irregular forms appropriately, for example 'went' and 'mice', as the phonological form had been more salient for him and less confusable than the regular forms. However, it was important to confirm for him that these were indeed the correct forms, and to prevent over-regularisation of the morphological endings that had been focused on.

Outcomes

Informal measures had been taken of William's progress through the therapy programme. For example, the accuracy of his identification of a given set of same/different non-word minimal pairs, such as /kɛp/, /tɛp/ and /mɔɪk/, /mɔɪt/, was recorded over successive presentations; a set of pictures illustrating words beginning with /k/ was presented for naming and the occurrences of /k/ rather than /t/ within these words noted. When increased awareness and usage of a particular contrast was observed, the next contrast was introduced. William did not achieve the use of such contrasts in all words but, for example, appropriate use of /k/ in naming pictures rose to 16 words out of 20 after 6 months of therapy (from a pre-therapy score of 5 out of 12 for correct use of /k/). Consistent across-word errors targeted in the therapy programme, and monitored in this way, included /k/ and /g/, /tʃ/, final consonants, /l/ and /s/ clusters. Progress was noted with each of these appearing more frequently in William's speech. However, auditory discrimination of minimal pairs and non-word pairs was somewhat unpredictable. This suggests that changes were effected in motor programmes, and possibly in phonological representations, but input processing difficulties persisted.

Unfortunately, no formal post-therapy testing was carried out, as transfer to another therapist took place quite quickly. However both therapist and teacher had reported that William's speech had become more intelligible over the period of therapy, and the production of words and phoneme contrasts that had been targeted in therapy improved. For example, he now articulated *rabbit* correctly and used /k/ and /g/ in most words appropriately. Syllable and initial and final conso- nant identification improved, and there was now some success in judging rhyme (scoring 11/12) although rhyme production was still not achievable. William still relied on orthographic representations for some phonological awareness tasks and was finding it difficult to separate the concept of the sounds of a word from the letters used to write it. Reading and spelling were showing some progress, although use of phonic strategies was still minimal. More recently his mother has reported a marked improvement in literacy skills. William showed more awareness and use of plural and past-tense endings, however use of these was not occurring in all appropriate contexts.

Therapy would have been best evaluated by:

- analysing further speech samples to examine where the consistent, across-word errors persisted
- assessing production of words targeted for word-specific errors
- carrying out tasks to examine whether discrimination of phonologi- cal distinctions and phonological representations were now more accurate.

The psycholinguistic assessment framework could also be utilised to re-profile William's speech processing skills, and to see what changes had occurred. It would be useful to feed back remaining speech errors in the auditory-visual lexical decision task, for example using a picture of a scooter, and asking 'Am I saying this word right?' followed by the correct version *scooter*, and William's pronunciation [sutə]. If he consistently accepts his own pronunciation as correct, this would suggest that his phonological representation for this word is still inaccurate. However, analysis of auditory discrimination skills would be required to ensure inaccurate responses were not the result of continuing input processing difficulties.

William's speech became more intelligible over the period of therapy. This was important in maintaining communication skills and confidence in situations that relied on verbal communication skills.

General implications

This case illustrates the interaction between auditory discrimination skills and the development of accurate phonological representations. A similar pattern of difficulty will be found in other children with Landau–Kleffner syndrome, and will also exist in some children with developmental speech and language disorders. The principle of using visual means to present phonological information and to update phonological representations is presented and examples of how this can be implemented are given. Using intact articulatory skills to say words correctly exploits bottom-up processing from motor execution to feed back phonological forms to the level of the motor programme and possibly also to the phonological representation (see Figure 1.2.3). The use of a psycholinguistic assessment framework (Stackhouse and Wells 1993, forthcoming) allowed the source of William's speech errors to be pinpointed and strengths and weaknesses in speech processing skills to be identified. This provided a clear rationale for therapy and ensured that the therapy programme was appropriate to the perceived processing deficits.

Acknowledgements

The author would like to express her gratitude to William for his perseverance, enthusiasm and sense of humour, which made it a pleasure to work with him. Thanks are also due to Roger Penniceard for allowing details from the psychological assessment to be used in this paper.

Chapter 1.3
Remediating auditory processing deficits in adults with aphasia

JULIE MORRIS

Many adults with acquired aphasia have difficulties understanding spoken language. It is assumed that different 'therapies' may be required, depending on the origin of the problem. However, this assumption is rarely tested in any kind of rigorous way, although it may be evident in the clinical setting. Howard and Hatfield (1987) suggest that

> Only if we know exactly *how* a particular treatment task is meant to affect *what* ability and *why* it does so, can therapy progress (p. 5).

It is clear that there is a need for a basic understanding of some of the core aspects of therapy – who, what, when and why. Byng and Black (1995) suggest that although an in-depth knowledge of the language deficit(s) is essential to therapy, it is insufficient alone. They also state that

> without theories about the process of therapy itself, the therapy will remain the missing link in developing a theory of change through rehabilitation (p. 314).

This chapter is an attempt to address some of these issues for one type of language disturbance. It presents a very specific therapy, focusing on language-deficit. The therapy used is not novel and will have been used by many clinicians working both with adults with acquired language problems and with children. Neither are the patients described particularly pure types of cases, both having mixed deficits. Two adults with acquired language problems, JAC and JS, are presented. Both had auditory processing deficits, but showed different patterns of breakdown when their performance was studied in detail. Both patients had more difficulty accessing information presented in the auditory modality than the written modality. However, they both had some problem accessing semantic information regardless of modality of presentation. Both patients took part in essentially the same therapy, although there were differences as their progression through therapy was dictated by their own performance.

The ability to understand spoken language is a complex process and it is clear that there are several potential underlying causes of the impairment (see Franklin 1989 for a discussion). The focus in this paper will be on difficulties perceiving and discriminating speech stimuli, which is often referred to as **word sound deafness**. This type of word deafness has also been referred to in the literature as **pure word deafness** (Denes and Semenza 1975) and **auditory verbal agnosia** (Schuell 1953). The patient's hearing is within normal limits or at least not grossly impaired. The deficit is thought to be a deficit of speech perception, and therefore differs from auditory agnosia in that the patient does not have problems recognising or identifying environmental sounds.

When patients are having difficulty discriminating speech, one possible source of assistance for the patient's comprehension is the use of lip-reading information. It is important however to remember that no phonemes are uniquely specified by their visual characteristics, though they may be distinguished from certain other groups of phonemes. Lip-reading information therefore provides a useful but incomplete set of cues. The other cue which is potentially made available through lip-reading is timing, that is, a cue that the person is going to speak. In this paper we are not attempting to distinguish exactly what information the person gains from attending to the speaker's face, but it will consistently be referred to as **lip-reading**.

The fact that patients with word sound deafness have a problem discriminating speech sounds may additionally affect performance on auditorily presented language tasks other than discrimination. Franklin predicted that the patients' repetition would be at least as impaired as their discrimination, and this was borne out by data from ES, the word sound deaf patient she reported. In fact, most patients described in the literature have some kind of output difficulty.

What effect a problem in discriminating phonemes has in terms of recognising or understanding spoken words remains unresolved. Luria (1970) argued that what he termed the **phonemic deficit**, in patients described as having sensory or Wernicke's aphasia, meant that patients could not understand spoken words because of the difficulty they had discriminating between similar phonemes. However, there is still debate about the nature of the relationship between auditory discrimination abilities and actual comprehension abilities of auditorily presented words. Caramazza *et al.* (1983) reported a patient who had 'a selective impairment in phonetic processing of acoustic signals' and hypothesised that this should result in a severe difficulty with auditory comprehension as

if the acoustic input cannot be processed adequately at a perceptual level, subsequent more abstract stages of processing (such as lexical access) will be affected and comprehension will be impaired (p. 141).

Franklin also predicted that if there was a severe problem in speech analysis, performance on all auditory comprehension tasks would be impaired. However, if the problem was mild she suggested context would be used to aid understanding, unless the task required accurate knowledge of incoming phonology. She described a patient, ES, who had word sound deafness, and was extremely impaired at tasks of phoneme discrimination and auditory lexical/semantic tasks. The conclusion is that because ES's discrimination problems were severe he was unable to use context to assist him in auditory semantic tasks.

Baker *et al.* (1981) suggested that the relationship is dependent on the level of difficulty of the task, so that if there are increased demands on phonological processing semantic errors increase, and in contrast increased semantic processing leads to increased phonological errors. In their study, patients with Wernicke's aphasia made more errors in a CVC identification task where the choice was two phonologically related pictures (e.g. pear–bear) than they did in discriminating the same items in an auditory same-different judgement. Additionally, in both the CVC identification task and in an auditory word-picture matching task with both semantic and phonological distracters, they made fewer errors with items where the foil was two distinctive features different from the target than one distinctive feature. Baker *et al.* claim, therefore, that the subject must be responding to the visual input in some kind of phono-logical way (rather than merely semantic). So, problems with discrimi-nation did manifest themselves in a semantic task, although in fact the majority error type on the word-picture matching test was semantic. The suggestion of Baker *et al.* was that when phonological processing was most difficult, semantic processing was affected.

Little has been written regarding therapy for auditory processing deficits in adults. Naeser *et al.* (1986) discussed the use of what they termed a 'sentence level auditory comprehension' treatment programme which aimed to train the patients 'to focus on verbal mat-erial without visual cues'. Therapy began with a fairly standard CVC discrimination task, and moved on to the patient identifying from a selection of 3–4 written words the one which he or she heard within a sentence, with the sentence frame becoming increasingly complex. In the group discussed, 5 of the 7 patients improved following therapy on the Token Test (Spreen and Benton 1977), a test of auditory compre-hension involving highly structured sentences with minimal variance in semantic load. The therapeutic approach reported by Gielewski (1989) is also of relevance here, though it gives few details of individuals' responses to treatment. The therapy was designed for patients who had what is described as a 'phonemic hearing impairment'. It worked through a hierarchy of levels where the discrimination involved became progressively more difficult, and where the amount of visual informa-tion was manipulated. This was done at quite an explicit level, with the use of mouth drawings to illustrate to the patients the type of sound they heard.

Investigations

Lengthy assessment was carried out with both patients (JAC and JS), and some of these assessment results will be discussed in order to form a complete picture of their language skills. However, it is their ability to deal with auditory information that is the primary focus here. Results for the two patients are presented in parallel, though there were occasions where, for various reasons, only one of them did a particular test.

General background

Patient 1, JAC, was a retired school teacher. At the time assessment began he was 61, and 8 months post-onset. However, the bulk of the results are from the period between 1 year 4 months post-onset and 1 year 8 months post-onset, when therapy began. A CT scan showed involvement of the anterior parietal region.

On initial presentation it was clear JAC was having a great deal of difficulty understanding what was being said to him. In response to a question he tended to produce jargon, with the occasional relevant item embedded in it. When encouraged, he would attempt to write down key items from his message, and this was by far the most successful form of communication for him. He had problems understanding instructions for tasks, and in the initial stages of testing had some problems moving between tasks, tending to perseverate earlier response types. Perseveration also occurred on individual items. Prior to involvement in this study, JAC had been having regular speech and language therapy which had included work on both auditory and written comprehension abilities, with the emphasis being on his auditory skills.

Patient 2, JS, was 73 and retired when he suffered his stroke, having worked as a tailor. A CT scan showed multiple large areas of low attenuation throughout the white matter of both cerebral hemispheres, with several areas of very low attenuation in the region of the left basal ganglia. He was 8 months post-onset when the work with him began, and 13 months post-onset when the actual therapy started. On a functional everyday level JS's communication consisted largely of social conversation such as greetings and requests for objects present in the immediate environment. When asking him for information, the use of yes/no type questioning elicited more information than any other means, but it was often clear he did not understand what was being said to him, and conversations were usually limited to the here and now. He made good use of gesture and facial expression to convey his message.

Tests of hearing and environmental sounds

Both patients' hearing was tested using an audiometer in their homes (i.e. with some background noise) and a threshold calculated by averaging over 500, 1000 and 2000 Hz. JAC's hearing was slightly impaired with a mean of 30 dB. This was not considered significant given that he was tested in ambient noise. JS's hearing was within normal limits with a mean threshold of 20 dB.

Both patients performed within normal limits on a test of environmental sound discrimination, each making only one error in a total of 20 items. In this task, they heard a sound (e.g. cat miaowing) and had to select from three pictures the one which corresponded to the sound. Of the two distracters one was unrelated and the second was either a similar sound (e.g. baby crying) or from a similar category of item (e.g. dog barking).

Speech sound discrimination tasks

To begin with, their ability to perceive fine differences between auditory stimuli will be discussed. On standard minimal pair testing, JAC performed reasonably. These are tasks traditionally used such as those in the ADA Comprehension Battery (Franklin *et al*. 1992) or in PALPA (Kay *et al*. 1992), where two CVC items are presented (words or non-words), which are either the same or where one phoneme has been altered, generally by one or two distinctive features, for example, *bit–bit* vs. *bit–pit*. The subject has to judge whether the pair are the same or different. On these kinds of tasks, JAC was almost always within the normal range, and his level of performance on examples of this type of task is shown in Table 1.3.1.

Table 1.3.1 Discrimination of CVC pairs (% correct)

	JAC	JS	Elderly normal range
Word strings e.g. cap–tap	97	62	82–100 (mean = 98.7)
Non-word strings e.g. dæk gæk	100	58 58 (FV) 70 (LR)	95–100 (mean = 99.5)
'Maximal' pairs using non-word strings e.g. tʌs gʌp	100	58 63 (FV) 92 (LR)	98–100 (mean = 99.6)

LR = lip-reading presentation; FV = free voice presentation.

In contrast, the second patient, JS, had great difficulty with these tasks. Asked to discriminate two CVC words, he was able to do so correctly for only 62% of the items. His performance was similar if the items were non-words, with a 58% success rate. His performance was also poor on a test where the contrasts to be discriminated were not all changes of only one or two distinctive features. A test was administered where the difference between the items to be discriminated varied from one phoneme changing by one distinctive feature (e.g. /peb/ – /ped/) to items where the two CVC pairs bore no resemblance to each other, both consonants differing by three distinctive features, and the vowel having changed (e.g. /gæb/ – /sʌs/). This will be referred to as the test of **maximal pairs**. For a full description of the test and items see Morris *et al.* (1996). On this he appeared to be having as much difficulty as in the previously described discrimination tasks, being correct on only 58% of the items. However, a clear pattern of errors emerged where JS was able to discriminate the items reliably if the change between the pairs made them sufficiently distinct. He made no errors for the items which bore no resemblance to each other (the /gæb/ – /sʌs/ example mentioned earlier), and began to make some errors with the less different items, making the most errors on pairs where the difference was small. JAC made no errors on this task, which is not surprising given how good he was at the standard discrimination tasks involving only one or two distinctive feature changes.

As mentioned above, lip-reading information is one source of possible assistance to patients such as JS. He was therefore reassessed on some of the tasks, varying the mode of presentation. Normally assessments were presented from tape over headphones, so that no cues were available. Speech was recorded on to a computer and digitised, with the aim of removing potential cues such as intensity differences or pitch differences. For JS, taped presentation was contrasted with two other modes of presentation referred to here as lip-reading and free voice.

- **Lip-reading presentation** means the patient was asked to look at the experimenter before an auditory stimulus was presented, so that he could pick up any cues to, for example, place of articulation, from lip and mouth position.
- **Free voice presentation** means that the patient was asked to look down, for example by focusing on the written or picture choice in front of him, so that this information was no longer available.

Contrasting these three modes of presentation meant it was possible to examine whether additional cues were being utilised to assist performance. This then might be of relevance in therapy.

JS was significantly helped if he was allowed to use lip-reading information in these discrimination tasks. His performance on the maximal pairs test improved to 92% correct in the lip-reading condition, a significant improvement over both tape presentation and over free voice presentation, where he was 63% correct (McNemar, free voice vs. lip-reading presentation, $p < 0.01$.). The same trend was seen in the non-word minimal pair performance with his score moving to 70% with lip-reading compared with 58% with free voice. However, this difference only approaches significance (binomial, $p = 0.062$). JAC's performance was not assessed contrasting lip-reading presentation with other presentation modes since his performance was close to ceiling with taped presentation. However, in situations where lip-reading information was potentially available to him, he did not choose to use it and did not naturally focus on the speaker's face.

So, from the results presented so far, it appears JS had a great deal of difficulty discriminating CVC items from each other, whereas JAC was well within normal limits. However, when the complexity of the task was increased, for example with strings longer than CVC items, JAC did begin to have some difficulty. Two tasks were developed which used longer strings (5–8 phonemes) taken from existing lexical decision tests. One used both words and non-words (e.g. *dungeon–dungeod*), and the other purely non-word strings (e.g. *baggle–bakkle*). JAC found both of these difficult, although he performed well above chance, getting 81–83% of items correct. Although older control subjects do make some errors, JAC was outside their range of performance (92–100% correct). Neither of these tasks was attempted with JS, as he had had such problems with the shorter CVC discrimination.

Tasks requiring lexical/semantic access

Following this, both patients were assessed on a range of tasks designed to look at their ability to access lexical and semantic information. The purpose was to look at the possible impact of their discrimination difficulties on other auditorily presented tasks. Written versions of the tasks were also presented to allow for comparison of spoken versus written presentation. The fact that JAC had some kind of problem processing auditory stimuli was confirmed by his performance on both lexical and semantic tasks, where he consistently had more difficulty with auditory than written presentation. On the ADA test of lexical decision where word and non-word items are presented, and the subject has to decide if the items are real words or not, JAC had no difficulty if the items were presented in a written form. However, with auditory presentation he had some difficulty, getting 81% correct. The normal error range for elderly controls is 91–99%.

The advantage of written over auditory presentation was again seen in semantic tasks, although here JAC was no longer within the range of normal performance, even with written presentation. As can be seen in

Table 1.3.2, in the ADA test of synonym judgements, JAC had difficulty with the task in both forms of presentation. This is a task where he heard or saw two words and had to judge if they had a similar meaning or not. When the pair were presented for him to read, he made 16 errors, with the older normal range being 0–10 errors. However, with auditory presentation he had much more difficulty, making 31 errors (older normal range = 1–14). This difference between modality of presentation is significant (McNemar, $p < 0.02$). This advantage for written presentation is also seen in a word-picture matching task. In this he saw four pictures: the target, and three distracters. One of the distracters was either semantically or phonologically related to the target, and the other two distracters were unrelated to the target, but related to each other. For example a target of *bridge* has a phonological distracter of *fridge*, and two unrelated distracters of *tie* and *tiger* (phonologically related to each other). JAC made only 2 errors when the target was written but 10 when presentation was auditory. The latter score is outside the normal range, where normals make 0–6 errors, with a mean error of 1. This difference between auditory and written presentation is significant (binomial, $p < 0.01$).

Table 1.3.2 Comparison of auditory vs. written presentation (expressed as percentage correct)

	Number of items	JAC		JS	
		Auditory	Written	Auditory	Written
ADA lexical decision	160	81	99	67	83
ADA synonym judgement	160	81	90	62	68
ADA word–picture match	66	85	97	71	80

JS also performed better on the lexical decision task when the same items were presented written as opposed to spoken. However, although better, he remained outside the normal level of performance, even with written presentation, making correct lexical decisions for 83% of items when they were written down (older normal mean = 99%; range = 94–100%). Even though he is outside the normal range, JS is still significantly better than when those same items were spoken, where he was correct only 67% of the time (McNemar, $p < 0.01$).

Similarly, JS appeared to show an advantage for written presentation of the semantic tests. However, the differences between auditory and written versions of these tests failed to reach significance. This is basically because JS had greater difficulty, and his scores with written presentation fell to a similar level to scores with auditory presentation. Table 1.3.2 details both patients' results.

The synonym judgement task described contrasts high imageability pairs (e.g. marriage–wedding) with low imageability pairs (e.g. truth–reality). JS made more errors on low imageability pairs when the items were written. He made 17 errors to low, versus 5 to high imageability pairs ($p < 0.01$), but showed no effect of imageability when the items were spoken. This confirms the notion of him having a central difficulty with semantics regardless of modality of presentation. The fact that there is no effect of imageability with spoken presentation is presumably because his additional auditory difficulties would mask any such effect.

JAC and JS were also tested on one measure of sentence comprehension, the Test for Reception of Grammar (TROG, Bishop 1982) which was presented auditorily. Both had considerable difficulty with the task, JAC scoring 42% correct and JS 56%. Both patients are therefore having difficulty processing auditory material. For JAC this is in contrast to relatively good performance when the same items are presented in written form. JS shows an advantage for written presentation in lexical decision, and a non-significant trend in tasks where he is required to access semantic information.

Tasks of repetition

JAC also had some difficulties in repetition. As Table 1.3.3 shows, on the ADA word repetition task, with high and low frequency, high and low imageability, and long and short words, he was able to reproduce 77% of the items correctly. His errors were mainly phonological (78% of errors) and his remaining responses were unrelated non-words or failure to make any attempt. Table 1.3.3 also shows the results of a repetition task which included both words and non-words. In this JAC was able to produce 53% of the words correctly, but only 23% of the non-words correctly. These non-words closely resembled words. The test included a set of non-words ('invented' non-words) which did not closely resemble any word, but were phonotactically plausible. He was completely unable to repeat any of these non-words. For all three types of stimuli, JAC's predominant error type was again phonological. Phonological errors here are any attempt where the response shares 50% of its phonemes with the target or viceversa. JAC was more likely to produce a phonological error for the word items than the non-words, and least likely for the 'invented' non-words, where he was almost as likely to produce an unrelated non-word response.

Repetition was extremely difficult for JS, and he was almost unable to repeat any items correctly; words or non-words. In the mixed repetition task he repeated 5 words correctly, and only 1 non-word. In the word repetition task he repeated only 1 item correctly, out of the 80 items presented. The fact that his errors are nearly all unrelated responses (90%

of his errors on the word repetition task) may be due to the severity of his impairment in auditory discrimination. The same sound string produced as an error for one item often reappeared as the response to an item later, although in a slightly different form, for example, for *hospital* JS produced /moskjul/, and then later for *cube* produced /mekjul/.

Table 1.3.3 Performance on repetition tasks (expressed as percentage correct)

	Number of items	JAC	JS
ADA word repetition	80	77	1
Mixed word and non-word repetition	160	29	4
Words		53	8
Non-words		23	2
Non-words not like words		0	0

Other tasks requiring spoken output

The patients' reading and naming abilities will now briefly be considered to provide some further background. JAC was able to read 66% of the words from the ADA oral reading test correctly. His errors were again predominantly phonological errors, and the remainder were productions of unrelated words, neologisms, and some perseverative responses. JAC had a great deal of difficulty reading non-words, and was unable to produce any correctly. The majority of his errors (45%) were unrelated to the target, and included some perseverations.

JAC's naming of the 60 items in the PALPA frequency naming test was also impaired. He named significantly more correctly when asked to produce the written name than when asked to produce a spoken name (McNemar, $\chi^2 = 7.68$, $p < 0.01$), producing a correct spoken name for 38% of items compared with 62% if written. When producing a spoken name, he frequently perseverated an earlier response (43% of his errors). As JAC has problems with all spoken output it seems likely that his impaired repetition ability was not due solely to input processing problems.

Contrasting JS's performance on these three tasks involving spoken output (word reading, non-word reading and picture naming), his performance was similar to his repetition, with him having great difficulty with all of the tasks. Only 28 of the 80 items from the ADA word reading task were actually attempted, as he found the task so difficult and was unable to produce any items correctly. Neither was he able to read any non-words. He also found it extremely hard to produce the names of pictures, correctly naming only 1 of 16 pictures attempted, and managing to correct himself on 1 other. In both reading and naming, as in repetition, all of his errors were unrelated to the target, and he tended to reproduce earlier errors, that is to perseverate his incorrect responses. For example, /til/ appeared as an initial response for *glass* and for *coke*. This all confirms that JS had a severe problem in producing spoken words, and that like JAC, his difficulty with repetition was not solely due to his poor auditory discrimination, although of course, in both patients, this may have contributed.

Baselines

Although both patients were assessed a considerable time post-onset, it could still be argued that there was some degree of spontaneous recovery taking place, or that their performance on language tests might vary for reasons other than the therapy. See Byng and Coltheart (1986) for a discussion of these issues. To eliminate these possibilities in order to be confident that any change seen after therapy was due to the therapy itself, both patients repeated a selection of the tests before therapy started, to establish that they showed a stable level of performance. The results are presented in Table 1.3.4.

Table 1.3.4 Repeated measures prior to therapy

	Maximum	*1*	*2*	*3*	*Time gap (months)*
Patient 1: JAC					
ADA auditory synonyms	160	129	131	130	2
Mixed repetition	160	41	46		6
ADA word reading	80	53	54		1
Patient 2: JS					
ADA auditory synonyms	160	100	102		3
Non-word discrimination	40	23	25		5

Both JS and JAC repeated the auditory synonym judgement test (JAC three times), and neither showed any significant change between administrations. For a variety of reasons the other tasks they repeated were different. JS repeated a discrimination task using non-words (different from the one discussed earlier) and scored 23 and 25 out of 40 respectively. JAC repeated the mixed repetition task and the word reading task, and both showed stable performance. On the repetition he scored 41 and then 46 out of 160 with a 6 month gap (McNemar, non significant) and on the word reading he scored 53 and 54 out of 80 respectively, with a 1 month gap, immediately prior to the therapy period. The conclusion was that prior to the therapy period both patients' performance on a variety of language tests was stable.

Therapy

Aims and assumptions

Both patients had difficulties processing auditorily presented input, in particular discriminating similar sounding items, and it was decided that this would be the focus of therapy. Improving their ability to discriminate speech sounds might improve their ability to understand spoken language in a more general sense. However, as discussed, the extent to which these discrimination problems impact on the ability to access lexical/semantic information is still unclear. It was also of interest to examine whether improving input skills had any effect on their output. It seems this could occur for two potential reasons. The first is simply that if the person is more accurate in perceiving the correct input, then they might be more accurate in reproducing the correct output. The second possibility is that they become better at monitoring their own output through improved auditory skills, thereby recognising their errors.

Therapy for the two patients was identical in as many respects as was possible, to allow evaluation of the same therapeutic approach with two different subjects. The notion was that rather than varying both the nature of the therapy and the nature of the kind of language deficit shown (i.e. a different patient), therapy content would remain constant and it would be the exact nature of the language deficit which would vary. As discussed above, both patients had auditory processing problems, but their profiles of difficulty were very different. Therapy for both patients consisted of twice weekly therapy over a 6 week period, that is 12 sessions in total. It is not clear what the optimum number of sessions per week would be. Twice weekly was chosen for several reasons including practicalities of fitting the sessions into a working week, and how much contact the patients (and their families) actually wanted. However, it was felt important that contact was more than once weekly, so that progress could be built upon.

Therapeutic tasks

Several task formats were chosen for use in therapy, but all had this same basic underlying aim of improving discrimination skills. As the therapy sessions were going to involve quite intensive listening it was felt vital to have some variety. Both patients responded favourably to the sessions, and sessions lasted between 40 minutes and an hour.

The therapy tasks used a variety of stimuli: consonant (+ schwa), CV and VC syllables, and CVC words. There were three kinds of discrimination task requiring a same/different judgement. Consonant discrimination was used, where two phonemes were presented auditorily (in reality this has to be the phoneme + the schwa vowel, e.g. /kə/) and the subject had to judge whether the same sound was presented on both occasions or not. The other two discrimination tasks involved discrimination of either CV or VC syllables. In the first, a pair of CV stimuli was presented, e.g. /ta/–/ka/, and the subject had to judge if they were the same or different. VC discrimination was exactly the same as the CV discrimination task, except that the consonant was final in the syllable, e.g. /ap/–/ab/. Same/different judgements with CVC stimuli were not used in therapy simply to avoid overuse of the assessment format.

An auditory to written word judgement task was also used. In this, one written word was presented and then a word was spoken. The subject had to judge if what was said matched what was written or not. Use of tasks with written choices meant a wide variety of words could be used, in contrast to word–picture tasks which are restricted to picturable (highly imageable/concrete) items. JAC had performed well with written stimuli in assessment so the use of written stimuli in these therapy tasks had the potential of supporting his problematic auditory processing. This was also true to some extent for JS, who had shown an advantage for written presentation, except where semantic access was required, which is not the case in these therapy tasks.

The final task type involved choosing the target (i.e. the word they heard) from an array before them, where two or three distracter items were included. The choice was either pictures (auditory word–picture matching) or words (auditory–written word matching). The third and final task of this type was a consonant identification task. In this, the patient was shown a choice of written letters (either 2 or 3) and one of them was then presented auditorily. The subject had to point to which letter had been said (i.e. phoneme + schwa, e.g. /kə/). JAC found this task extremely difficult on his first and only time of doing it, basically performing at chance. As it was only a means of practising his discrimination skills, instead of proceeding with a task he was at chance at, a slightly easier version of the task was introduced for him which was a phoneme–grapheme judgement task. A phoneme (+ the schwa vowel) was presented auditorily and the corresponding grapheme presented orthographically. JAC simply had to decide whether what he saw and what he heard matched or not. He clearly still found the task difficult, taking a long time, but he was able to perform above chance.

In all tasks the emphasis was on listening skills, and response load was kept to a minimum. For all tasks the only response actually required was to point, either to their choice from the array of stimuli, or if the decision was whether the items were the same or different, then 'same' and 'different' were written down. If they chose either to repeat what they heard or to read written choices this was neither encouraged nor discouraged. However, if their attempt was incorrect then the correct word was said, but there was no indication given that they should re-attempt. This was merely so that they heard the correct model.

Feedback during therapy

The kind of feedback given during therapy was felt to be a crucial aspect of therapy. Emphasis was placed on the patient being aware of his performance, and being aware that the therapy sessions were different from assessment. It is possible that, with a highly structured set of tasks such as those used here, the patients could feel they were simply doing more assessment. To begin with, the division between assessment and therapy was discussed with the patients and their families. A detailed record was kept of performance on tasks during the therapy sessions. However, to avoid the patient being very aware of his performance being scored, an audio tape was made of the complete session, and scoring done later from this.

In the assessment period no specific feedback had been given; that is the patients were never told if a specific item was correct or not. In contrast, within therapy, feedback was given immediately on every item so that the patient knew if he had been successful or not. If they were correct, they were told so, and they moved on to the next item. If incorrect, again they were told so, and the item was repeated, if possible reducing the complexity slightly. This was done by changing the mode of presentation, so that if the item was presented initially in a free voice mode and they were incorrect, on repetition of the item, it would be presented with lip-reading. If still incorrect, then the correct answer was given. The answer would then be repeated, asking the subject to look (i.e. encouraging them to use lip-reading information) and **cued articulation** (Passy 1990) was used to highlight the relevant sound contrast.

Cued articulation is a system of small hand-signs designed to give visual information about individual phonemes. Each phoneme is represented by a unique hand sign, with signs having elements in common with each other, as do phonemes themselves. So, for example, the phoneme /p/ is represented by the thumb and forefinger being held together at the side of the mouth (the placement of the sound) and then they move apart rapidly representing the plosive nature of the sound (the manner). To differentiate it from its voiced counterpart /b/, /p/ uses just a single finger to denote that it is voiceless. In contrast, when signalling the phoneme /b/ with cued speech, both the middle and forefinger are used. This use of two fingers consistently marks voicing in the other phonemes. This system was felt to be highly useful as a means of providing visual information representing an auditory distinction the patients were having difficulty hearing. The use of this system was not discussed in detail with either patient, as it was not felt appropriate to discuss detailed phonemic information with them because of their poor comprehension. The hand-signs were introduced in the feedback and lay-terms were used to accompany the cues, such as describing voiced sounds as 'noisy', compared with 'quiet' voiceless sounds. The system was not taught but simply used as required, as a means of providing additional cues for the patients to use if they found them helpful.

Four tasks were used every session, using both lip-reading and free voice presentation modes. A task was introduced in a session with lip-reading encouraged and then the task was continued or completely repeated with free voice presentation.

Design of therapy

The complexity of therapy was manipulated in three ways which it was hoped would gradually increase the level of difficulty. These were phonemic similarity of the items and their distracters, presentation mode, and number of distracters. With JS, assessment had shown that he had a great deal of difficulty discriminating similar sounding items, although he was able to discriminate items if they were sufficiently distinct. This therefore gave a possible starting point for therapy, beginning with differences he was able to perceive reliably, and gradually, moving through the sessions, items to be discriminated, or targets and their foils became more similar, in terms of the phonemic difference between them. In this way therapy began at a level where JS could be successful to some degree. JAC, as discussed, was unimpaired at the maximal pairs task (although did have some minor problems with other minimal pair tasks), and so, given that there was no indication from assessment of where to begin with JAC as there had been with JS, therapy with JAC began at the same point. There was no measure taken of acoustic similarity, which may of course affect the difficulty of the task. That is, items that differ in the same way phonemically might actually be very different in terms of their acoustic similarity.

The second manipulation within the tasks was mode of presentation. Assessment had shown that the presence or absence of lip-reading information affected JS's chance of success. Therefore tasks were initially presented with lip-reading, and then later with free voice presentation, so that the patient had to rely on auditory cues alone. As other subtle cues (unwittingly given by the speaker) could still be operating with free voice presentation (for example, different presentation rates or volume for different than for same pairs), in the latter sessions, the items were presented on tape over headphones, as had been done in assessment. The final way that complexity was manipulated was by the number of distracters present in the matching tasks. Initially two distracters were used, moving to three. The effect of the number of distracters had not been clearly demonstrated in assessment, but one distracter was used initially on the basis of keeping the task requirements as simple as possible, and then two, to move away from a decision where there was a 50% chance of getting the item correct.

JAC and JS's progression through therapy

Therapy was planned systematically in this way prior to its commencement. However, progress in the session was closely monitored so that if the patient found particular difficulty with a certain level or a certain task, then subsequent plans were modified accordingly. This has already been pointed out for JAC, where consonant identification was not used as he scored at chance on this task. The tasks were only vehicles for the aim of therapy, and therefore were to be adapted according to the patient's response to them. There would be no purpose in the patient consistently failing a task when other ways of practising phonemic discrimination could be utilised. If, however, the patient scored above chance but was still making errors, it would be assumed this was to do with the level of difficulty rather than just simply the task, and so more practice would be given at this level. The criterion for moving on was 80% or more correct. It was felt that more than 80% would be too strict a criterion, because of lapses in concentration for instance, and to ensure a steady progression through the stages described. If they were below this level, the task was repeated in subsequent sessions, or different items used but without a change in difficulty, until they reached the 80% criterion. In this way it was hoped that they would achieve a reasonable feeling of success, whilst being challenged by some of the therapy items.

Table 1.3.5 details JAC's and JS's progression through therapy by task and by session. This allows us a broad overview of the levels of success for each patient on the different tasks, and also demonstrates that not only were they dissimilar in their initial profile, but that this was reflected in their response to therapy, session by session.

As Table 1.3.5 shows, therapy proceeded as planned for the majority of tasks and sessions for JAC. Not surprisingly, he had little difficulty initially, only beginning to have difficulty in session 9 (where only one consonant differed by one distinctive feature), where he did not reach the 80% success criterion on the auditory–written word matching task, and therefore he did not move on in terms of the next stage or level of difficulty (on that task). The one exception in this progression was the phoneme–grapheme judgement task on which JAC only once reached the criterion. It would seem clear that there was something additionally difficult in this task for JAC beyond the discrimination involved, and perhaps this was not a particularly useful task to include.

As can be seen in Table 1.3.5, JS's performance was much more irregular, and he had difficulties from the earliest sessions on at least some of the tasks despite the fact that therapy began with a discrimination he had been shown to be able to do in assessment. Due to this, the progression through the different 'levels' did not proceed as planned for JS. He moved forward (in terms of phonemic difference) in some tasks, but not others. On those tasks where he did not reach the 80% criterion, he remained at the same 'level' for the next session, and so on.

Table 1.3.5 Progression through therapy sessions (expressed as percentage correct on the different tasks)

Patient 1: JAC		Session number											
		1	2	3	4	5	6	7	8	9	10	11	12
A	LR		(50)		80	**68**		76	72				**68**
A	FV				**76**	**60**		**60**	**60**				**52**
B	LR	100		100			100		100				
B	FV	100		92			96		92			**98**	**94**
C	LR	96	96	92	96	100	100	92	92	92	96	**86***	**96***
C	FV	100	92	92	100	**84**	96	96	88	92	96		
D	LR		90	92		92				88	88		
D	FV			80		92				96	92		
E	LR	92	92						**88**	92	**72**		**100**
E	FV	92	84						**84**	**72**	**76**	**74**	**72**
F	LR			100	96		100	100		100		**96***	
F	FV			100	100		96	96		100		100	
G	LR				96	100	100		100		100		**80***
G	FV				100	100	100		96		**88**		**88**

Patient 2: JS		Session number											
		1	2	3	4	5	6	7	8	9	10	11	12
A	LR	77	70			**76**	**82**	**65**	**71**	**65**			
A	FV	77	67			**70**	**53**		**24**	**65**			**53**
B	LR		75	64	81						**96**		
B	FV			84	77						**96**	**	
C	LR	100	96	92	85	81				**81***	**73***	**64***	**
C	FV	100		81	85		**62**	**69**	**59**	**65***			
D	LR	94	80		96		**72**						**70***
D	FV	98			68		**88**					**	
E	LR			68		84		**68**	**88**	**58***	**64***	**58***	**72***
E	FV			84		80		**64**	**72**				
F	LR					**62**	**90**				**92***		
F	FV						**75**			**87**			
G	LR							**85**				**75***	**80***
G	FV							**60**	**70**				

Codes for the tasks:

A   phoneme–grapheme identification
B   consonant discrimination
C   auditory word–picture matching
D   auditory–written word judgment
E   auditory–written word matching
F   CV discrimination
G   VC discrimination
LR = lip-reading presentation; FV = free voice presentation
* = task presented on tape
( ) = Original task (i.e. phoneme–grapheme matching) before modified for JAC
Bold = tasks where patient did not reach criterion
** = task done, but no score available

Outcomes

Table 1.3.6 shows the results of pre- and post-therapy assessments for JAC and JS. It was hoped that the therapy focusing on JAC's ability to discriminate increasingly similar sounds would improve his performance on tasks believed to require this skill. However, no change was seen on either of the longer item discrimination tests repeated post-therapy. Other auditorily presented tasks also showed no change. The ADA tests of lexical decision and synonym judgement with auditory presentation both remained static. Both of these might have been expected to improve if his ability to process auditory stimuli had improved as a result of therapy. The only task for JAC which showed improvement was his ability to repeat items in the mixed word and non-word repetition task. Overall his ability to repeat items was significantly better (McNemar, $p < 0.01$). When looked at separately, JAC was significantly better at repeating real words (McNemar, $p < 0.02$) but not significantly better at repeating non-words although the trend was in the right direction. He continued to be unable to repeat any of the 'invented' non-words correctly. In contrast to this, on the other repetition task JAC did, which contained only real words, his performance did not change at all, his best score pre-therapy matching his post-therapy score exactly (77%). This may be because there was less room for improvement. JAC continued to make predominantly phonological type errors, as he had before therapy.

Table 1.3.6 Performance on a range of auditory tasks pre- and post-therapy (expressed as percentage correct)

Test	JAC Pre	JAC Post	JS Pre	JS Post
Word CVC minimal pairs			65	90
Non-word CVC min pairs			LR: 70	90
			FV: 57	80
Maximal pairs			Tape: 58	94
			FV: 62	79
Longer minimal pairs:				
Word and non-word	81	86		
Non-word only	83	86		
Auditory lexical decision	84	83	67	75
Auditory synonyms	82	81	64	72
Repetition (overall)	29	40		
Words only	53	75	1	12
Non-words only	23	32		
Invented non-words	0	0		
TROG	42	39	56	66
Word reading	66	65		

LR = lip-reading presentation; FV = free voice presentation.

In contrast to the improvement seen on the mixed repetition task, JAC's reading of single words showed no change following therapy. Prior to therapy he read 66% of the items correctly compared with 65% following therapy, which confirms that the improvement seen in his repetition was due to improvement in his processing of the auditory input rather than improvement in his spoken output skills which would have led to improvement in word reading as well.

The changes between JS's pre- and post-therapy performances will now be contrasted. As described earlier, unlike JAC, JS was impaired on a range of CVC discrimination tasks, and his performance on these improved significantly following the therapy period. The ADA test which requires discrimination of CVC words was repeated and a significant change was seen, from 65% correct at baseline testing to 90% correct after therapy (McNemar, $p < 0.01$). On the non-word discrimination task, the items were repeated in both free voice and lip-reading versions, so that the issue of whether lip-reading helped him could be examined further. With free voice presentation, JS improved significantly following therapy, from 57% to 80% (McNemar, $p < 0.05$). A similar trend was seen with lip-reading presentation, but this did not reach significance, presumably because he was closer to ceiling initially with lip-reading, so there was less room for improvement. In keeping with these results, his performance on the 'maximal' pairs test also showed significant change when the items were presented on tape (McNemar, $p < 0.001$) and this was replicated when the test was repeated with free voice presentation (binomial, $p < 0.011$). Performance with lip-reading presentation remained good, as it was pre-therapy. Following therapy, there was no significant advantage of lip-reading presentation over free voice, though there remained a trend (binomial, $p = 0.062$; non significant). See Table 1.3.6 for his scores on these tasks.

Other auditorily presented tasks were also repeated following the therapy period. Although therapy was not aimed at accessing lexical/semantic information from the auditory modality, improved ability to process auditory stimuli might affect his performance on other auditorily presented tasks. A trend of improvement was seen for his performance on auditory lexical decision, auditory synonyms and the TROG, but neither of these numerical changes reached statistical significance (see Table 1.3.6). Prior to therapy he had got 67% correct, and following therapy he got 75% correct on the ADA auditory lexical decision task, but this is a non-significant difference. Similarly on ADA auditory synonym judgements he shows a trend for improvement, moving from 64% correct at baseline, to 72% correct after therapy, but again this does not reach significance. On the TROG, he got 56% of items correct pre-therapy, compared with 66% following therapy, again a non-significant change. There was no such trend in JS's performance on written synonyms: on PALPA test of written synonyms, JS scored 63% after therapy, compared with 68% before.

Interestingly, as for JAC, JS's ability to repeat items did show significant improvement following the therapy period. Prior to therapy commencing, JS had correctly repeated only one item from a possible 80. Following therapy, this increased to 10 items correct. This is a significant change (binomial, $p = 0.012$). His ability to name pictures did not change significantly, with JS naming 2 items correctly after therapy compared with 1 before. As for JAC, this suggests the improvement seen in JS's repetition was due to improvements in his input processing rather than in his spoken output abilities.

JS's family reported they felt he had benefited from the therapy and paid more attention in conversations. JAC seemed to become more attentive in sessions as therapy progressed, and problems with shifting task and understanding task explanations appeared to decrease. However, no quantitative measures of functional improvement were taken, and so this cannot be commented upon further.

Discussion

An attempt has been made here to examine the efficacy of the same therapy programme used with two patients who had broadly similar problems. They both had auditory processing deficits, but detailed testing of their language revealed that there were fundamental differences. Assessment of JAC's language showed that he had problems with auditory processing tasks where lexical and semantic access was required, but difficulties with discrimination tasks arose only when the processing demands were increased. JS on the other hand, had problems with all auditorily presented tasks. Additionally, JS had difficulties with tasks requiring access to semantic information, irrespective of modality. So, the two patients had been shown to have qualitatively different auditory processing problems, and their response to therapy confirms this difference.

Post-therapy reassessment showed that, for both patients, therapy changed at least one aspect of their language performance. The only improvement in JAC's language abilities following this auditory discrimination work was in his ability to repeat words. For JS, his ability to discriminate between similar sounds improved dramatically. For both patients, effects were limited to tasks relevant to the focus of therapy, demonstrating that the improvements did not form part of some more generalised improvement but rather were a result of the specific content of therapy. Neither were they the result of more generalised recovery, demonstrated by the stability of the scores prior to therapy.

There was a suggestion that for JS improvement in discrimination ability had some effect on other tasks where auditory processing was required. There was a trend of improvement in auditory lexical decision and auditory synonym judgements and, like JAC, his ability to repeat words improved significantly. It should be remembered that JS had problems with tasks requiring access to semantic information even with written presentation, and therapy was not designed to address this central difficulty with semantics. JS's performance on auditorily presented semantic tasks would therefore not have been expected to approach ceiling as a result of therapy.

An important question arising is how was the improvement in JS's speech discrimination abilities possible? As has been shown, following therapy, JS's performance with free voice presentation on the CVC discrimination tasks approached that with lip-reading. This suggests that JS was actually better able to hear the differences between the phonemes post-therapy; it was not simply an effect of utilising the lip-reading information more effectively, although it is of course possible that this did occur at some point in the therapeutic process. The fact remains, however, that even without being able to see the speaker's face (and so use lip-reading information) JS's discrimination ability improved. He may in some sense have 'internalised' this skill. The cued articulation hand-signs may have drawn JS's attention to the type of contrasts which exist between phonemes. Perhaps he was helped to use the acoustic cues which were present and which had been, to some extent, made explicit during therapy. A second possible account is that his ability to attend to auditory stimuli improved, in some kind of general way, perhaps pointing to an attentional problem underlying the difficulty. These are only hypotheses which call for testing by further research.

Assessment of JAC's discrimination abilities had shown that he only failed when the degree of difficulty was increased, shown by his performance on the longer minimal pair tasks. He responded well to the therapy, moving forward through planned stages, consistently reaching the 80% success criterion, until the latter stages, where he did experience some difficulty with some of the tasks. Therapy therefore did suggest he was having some discrimination problems (even with CV and CVC stimuli) but it did not improve his performance on auditorily presented tasks (other than repetition). Perhaps JAC, whilst having some difficulty, was in fact not making sufficient errors on many of the auditory tasks to allow improvement to manifest itself in accuracy data.

Only his ability to repeat changed significantly for words, and there was a non-significant trend for non-words. There are several possible reasons for this. Possibly he may have improved his ability to attend to the close detail of auditory stimuli as a result of therapy, or his ability to monitor his own output may have improved. It is not possible to distinguish these possibilities from the data here.

One of the issues introduced earlier was the controversy which exists regarding whether a deficit in phoneme discrimination affects the ability to access lexical/semantic information when it is presented auditorily. Therapy studies with patients with auditory discrimination problems are one possible way of addressing this. It seems likely that if a person's auditory discrimination skills improve, and their scores on other auditorily presented tasks improve following discrimination work, then this reflects a common deficit rather than two separate deficits improving. JS's data support this to some extent, but are inconclusive. We see a trend of improvement in other auditorily presented tasks, but this only reaches significance with word repetition. There is a suggestion then that improving JS's ability to hear fine differences between speech sounds has improved his ability to access lexical/semantic information from the auditory modality, but it is not definitive, mainly because of JS's additional central semantic problem. One other consideration is that perhaps when we look at accuracy scores on auditory lexical/semantic tasks as a measure of improvement (as was done here), we are simply using too gross a measure. The other way improvement could potentially manifest itself is in the amount of processing time required for a task. Perhaps when the patient perceives the word accurately (following auditory discrimination therapy), and, if necessary, can complete the task without recourse to contextual information, the processing time required to access lexical/semantic information will be reduced. This is an issue for future research.

Many issues have been identified here which require further consideration. It is vital that we continue to study the therapeutic process in detail, and develop our understanding of what kind of therapy is effective for which patient and how, described by Byng and Black (1995) as 'the theory of therapy', and here, as the 'who, what, when and why'.

Acknowledgements

I am sincerely grateful to both JAC and JS and their families for allowing me to work with them, and for tolerating such extensive testing, and to Sue Franklin for comments on early drafts. I would like to thank speech and language therapists Debbie Lapin and Catherine Exley for referring JS to the project, and to Margaret Robinson for referring JAC and for her helpful discussions and time. Finally, I'd like to thank the neuropsychology group at York University for all their invaluable contributions.

Chapter 1.4
Afterword

SHULA CHIAT

The cases presented here share a common starting-point: impairment at the stage of auditory input processing. Both child and adult subjects evidenced difficulties in tasks which require auditory discrimination, in the absence of hearing impairment. For the adults, problems with auditory processing were also indicated by better performance with written than spoken input.

In the case of 10 year old William, whose problems set in when he was 3 years 6 months, difficulties at the stage of speech input processing might be expected to affect all subsequent stages of lexical and sentence processing. Such wider problems were indeed observed, though it is not clear how far these were attributable to constraints on William's auditory input. The fact that his repetition of words was superior to his naming suggests that he was perceiving distinctions that he had not stored. This could be because he had problems with lexical representations which went beyond constraints imposed by his auditory perception. On the other hand, his inferior naming could be a hangover from earlier difficulties with auditory perception which have left their mark in stored phonological representations.

In the adult cases, previously established representations might in principle be preserved, but access to them might be blocked by constraints on auditory input. It is also possible that such constraints could have a knock-on effect on subsequent stages of processing, even if these were not directly affected, or they might anyway be affected in their own right. The extensive assessments reported by Morris indicate that both patients had additional difficulties in language processing which were not entirely attributable to their perception. To different degrees, both showed difficulty with input tasks tapping lexical phonology, lexical semantics, and sentence comprehension, though for JAC difficulties were generally confined to the spoken modality. To different degrees, both also showed difficulty in output tasks including repetition, reading, and naming. Their performance on these assessments

points to problems in semantic representations and in output processing for which auditory processing could not be solely responsible. The
relations between the different levels at which difficulties were observed
are not, however, explored.

Although the psycholinguistic point of departure is similar in these
child and adult therapy studies, they diverge to some extent in their
approach to therapy. Therapy for the adult subjects targeted their auditory discrimination directly. Therapy tasks included same/different
judgements about auditorily presented word or non-word pairs, and
selection of pictures, written words or letters in response to auditory
stimuli. Auditory discrimination was, though, supported by the visual
cues of lip-reading and cued articulation. In post-therapy assessments,
JAC showed no improvement in auditory discrimination or in other
assessments of word or sentence processing apart from repetition. JS,
on the other hand, showed significant improvement in all auditory
discrimination tasks, even when visual cues were removed. He also
showed a trend towards better performance in auditorily presented
word and sentence assessments.

In William's case, therapy made explicit use of strengths to target
weaknesses in auditory discrimination. The visual modality was
exploited through lip-reading, cued articulation, and written forms with
coloured underlining of letters. In addition, speech output skills were
used to support sound and word contrasts William was having difficulty
perceiving, to enable him to update motor programmes based on inadequate discrimination. In its explicit use of visual cues and motor output
skills to support auditory discrimination, therapy could be seen as
working on connections between auditory processing and other levels
of processing rather than on auditory processing itself. Following
therapy, William showed improvement in his production of sounds and
words which had been targeted, and was reported by his therapist and
teacher to be more intelligible. His auditory discrimination, though,
remained unreliable.

So, we have one child showing improvement in his lexical output but
not in auditory discrimination; one adult showing virtually no improvement; and one adult improving in auditory discrimination and also in
processing lexical and sentence input. What can we infer from these
varying results of intervention? In making inferences, we must of course
bear in mind the many dimensions on which the individuals may differ:
the nature and extent of their difficulties in speech perception, the way
these difficulties affect their language processing more generally, their
attitude to their difficulties, their attitude to intervention, to name but a
few. Such differences could justify different approaches to intervention,
or explain different effects of the same intervention. In the face of these
potentially vast differences, certain observations about intervention and
its effects emerge from these cases.

First, therapy in all cases relied to some extent on strengths to overcome the weaknesses in speech discrimination. All drew on the visual modality, and in William's case, motor skills were also recruited. It would seem that, in order to tackle difficulties in auditory input, resorting to accessible cues to auditory differences is necessary. The different effects of these cues in each case suggest that there were differences in each individual's auditory processing deficit and its relation to other stages of processing. It appears that William could take advantage of the cues used to undo the repercussions of his auditory processing deficit, but that the deficit itself did not shift. This may reflect the resistence of auditory imperception to intervention. If a sound distinction cannot be 'perceived', perhaps there is no way of making it directly perceptible. In the case of JAC, who showed virtually no improvement, it is likely that the impairment in his auditory discrimination was so marginal that his progress in therapy tasks had no observable effects on assessments of discrimination or on most other aspects of processing. In contrast, the improvements shown by JS suggest that he was capable of discriminating more features of auditory input than he was actually discriminating, and that therapy alerted him to these features by providing him with indirect (visual) cues to them or by focusing his attention on them. To gain further insight into the outcomes of therapy for JAC and JS, we would perhaps need to know more about the source of their auditory discrimination difficulties and the relationship between their auditory processing and other aspects of lexical input and output processing.

The collective conclusions we might draw from these studies are:

- When we observe difficulties in auditory discrimination, we need to explore these in the context of the patient's wider lexical processing in order to identify which aspects of lexical processing are most spared/impaired.
- A patient may be capable of finer discrimination than he/she is achieving, so that focused listening – particularly aided by cues which are more accessible to that patient – may lead to improvements.
- A patient may be making maximum use of discrimination abilities, in which case practice alone will not effect change in auditory discrimination, but alternative cues may be used to support inadequate discrimination and so reduce its impact on other aspects of lexical processing.
- It may be that alternative cues can **circumvent** constraints on auditory discrimination or **strengthen** discrimination, but that they cannot **overcome** constraints, i.e. cannot make perceptible distinctions which were previously imperceptible.

That therapists turn to more intact dimensions of processing to bolster disrupted aspects is not surprising. In the introduction, we saw how this was happening with a variety of interventions for phonological impairment in children. In these interventions, it was intact input which was actively manipulated to drive changes in output. The challenge is to identify which **particular** strengths can be exploited effectively for which **particular** weaknesses. We might first look to an alternative modality, such as the visual modality, to make available distinctions which are blurred in the dominant modality, as in the use of lip-reading to support phonological discrimination. Then we might look for strengths in the impaired modality. Here we explore the possibility that a relatively intact level might support processing at a more impaired level. For example, discrimination between similar sounding words might be supported by highlighting their distinct semantics, or the difference in their motor production. Taking this approach, the more we understand about connections between different representations in processing, the more clues we have about how one aspect of a representation might be supported by another.

The focus of these studies on speech input is unusual in the field of psycholinguistically motivated therapy, and raises novel questions about the connections involved in input processing and the ways these may be exploited. Exploration of the nature and treatment of speech output processing has been more extensive, particularly in the developmental field, and has led to the elaboration of models of speech output (see Chapter 1.1). This has not been matched in the modelling of speech input. In identifying deficits of speech discrimination, these studies beg questions about what is involved in the gross processes of 'hearing' and 'speech discrimination', and how they intermesh. Vance touches on these issues at the outset of Chapter 1.2, when she points out that the auditory agnosia which William had earlier demonstrated had resolved, but that he might still have had difficulty with fine non-verbal auditory discrimination which was not tested. This leaves us wondering how William's deficit does or does not relate to hearing impairment. The same query arises for JAC and JS.

William's profile on speech assessments is also tantalisingly relevant to questions about the interaction between auditory input processing and the representation of phonological and semantic information about words. As we have seen, the superiority of his repetition over his naming shows that he was benefiting from hearing a model of a word, which means that he was hearing more distinctions than he had stored in his lexical representations. Paradoxically, though, his very poor repetition of non-words and his tendency to lexicalise them imply that his lexical representations were better specified than his auditory input. These data suggest that disrupted input affects the formation of representations but that previously formed representations aid the processing of input which is disrupted.

In order to throw more light on these stages of input processing and the ways in which they may be impaired, we might turn to the substantial research on normal speech perception. Going beyond a diagnosis of 'auditory discrimination problems' to a better understanding of the processes which integrate heard stimuli and relate them to semantic representations may give us new ways of thinking about how constraints on speech discrimination may be overcome.

Part 2
Lexical processing

Chapter 2.1
Introduction

JANE MARSHALL

Word finding problems are virtually ubiquitous in child and adult language disorder. However, their manifestation varies greatly. One obvious sign is hesitancy, as the person gropes for the desired word. Single word errors are a further sign. These can be grouped into broad categories, depending on their relationship to the target. For example, semantic errors are related in terms of meaning, while phonological errors are related in terms of sound. Real word errors which bear no obvious relationship to the target are often termed verbal paraphasias. some examples of these basic error types as shown in Table 2.1.1. Some apparent errors may reflect the person's attempt to compensate for their difficulties. For example, when stuck for the word *cactus*, some speakers may be able to say 'plant ... holly ... no'. These approximations are known to be wrong, but may at least direct the listener to the target. When evaluating errors, it is therefore important to take note of the person's awareness and intention in producing those errors.

Table 2.1.1 Basic error types

Target	Error	Type
camel	elephant	semantic
grass	glass	phonological
spanner	hammer	semantic/phonological
daffodil	solicitor	verbal paraphasia

In some cases of language disorder it is hard to believe that there are word finding difficulties. An example would be **jargon aphasia**, e.g.:

Experimenter: 'What is this' (target *telephone*)
Aphasic Person: 'oh that, that sir. I show you then what is a /'zæprɪks/ for the /'ɛlenkɒm/ with the /'pɪdlənd/ thing to th ... and then each of the /'pɪdləmz/ has an /'əɪjɪn/ on two three and so on and the /əedrnm/ can be correct to /sus/ taken. But it's a ... a thing of document.' (KC, Butterworth 1985)

This person does not obviously have a problem in accessing words, indeed there seems to be an **overgeneration** of speech, albeit often wrong. Yet instrumental analysis showed that this apparently fluent speaker was in fact hesitant, and that most of the hesitations occurred prior to errors. It seems that, even here, the speaker paused to seek the correct word and then replaced it with a neologism (Butterworth 1979).

An obvious early question is whether anomia reflects an absence of vocabulary, or a failure of access. Here the issues for adults and children are probably different. Investigations with adults suggest that most have problems of access. A number of factors lead to this conclusion. First, naming is often inconsistent, in that a word may be achieved on one occasion but not on another. Secondly, many adults can respond to cues. For example, providing information about the meaning of a word, or its initial sound will often prompt its production (see for example Howard and Orchard Lisle 1984, Bruce and Howard 1987). If words were lost to the system no amount of cueing would bring them back. Finally, there is the evidence that naming can be improved with therapy (see Nickels and Best 1996a, b for a review). Of course it is possible that such intervention has the effect of re-establishing lost lexical entries. However, a more likely account is that it helps to facilitate access, particularly when generalisations to untreated words occur.

The case for children is different. First of all, we must anticipate the normal developmental constraints on vocabulary acquisition. It would be quite unreasonable to expect a child of 6 to know words such as *existentialism* or *procurator fiscal*. Children with word finding difficulties may reveal additional immaturities of vocabulary, precisely because their processing disorder obstructs acquisition. Thus some of the word finding failures of these children may be due to an absence of vocabulary which we would normally expect to be present. Yet, these children also show problems in accessing words which **are** in their system. Here the presentation is similar to adults, in that we see inconsistency, hesitancy and the potential to respond to cues (see for example Chiat and Hunt 1993).

Another, linked question is whether some types of words are easier than others. Here the answer is clearly 'yes', although most evidence is drawn from studies with adults. One highly influential factor is the frequency or familiarity of the word, in that common words like *dog* are generally more accessible than uncommon ones like *ant*. Semantic properties are also important, in that concrete words are usually easier than abstract ones (Franklin *et al.* 1995). This is not surprising. However, very occasionally we encounter adults for whom the opposite is true, i.e. abstract words are favoured over concrete ones (see for example Warrington and Shallice 1984, Marshall *et al.* 1996). Age of acquisition may also be a factor, since the early words seem most robust even in adult aphasia (Morrison *et al.* 1992). Of course interpreting this finding is difficult, as this variable is likely to interact with other important factors, such as familiarity and concreteness. However, early words may have a particular semantic status, possibly because of their association with fundamental sensory motor experiences.

Word finding problems are not unique to language disorder. Virtually all of us experience occasional difficulties in thinking of the words we want to use. Furthermore, when this happens, the same general patterns emerge. Thus unimpaired speakers produce semantic and phonological errors and are sensitive to the same lexical properties as disordered speakers. For example, we know that 'normals' tend to hesitate before unusual words, suggesting that, just like aphasic people, they find these words difficult to access (Butterworth 1979).

What do word finding blocks tell us about how words are normally accessed? The existence of semantic and phonological errors suggests that word finding is not all or nothing, i.e. it seems possible to access some features of a word but not others. This, in turn, suggests that word production is accomplished in a number of 'stages', each of which can be impaired. We can represent these stages in the model shown in Figure 2.1.1. In the first stage of production the concept or idea accesses a word's **semantic representation**. This might be imagined as a cluster of features which makes up its meaning. Thus the features for *cat* might be: *animal, domestic, feline, fur, tail, whiskers* etc. The second stage accesses a **phonological representation**. It seems that this stage is heavily influenced by the word's frequency, in that very common words become available more readily than uncommon ones. The **output buffer** stores the word until it is required, and the final stage accesses the **motor programmes** for its production. The whole process might be envisaged as a cascade of activation from one level to the next. Thus at the semantic level all the features of *cat* are activated to a point at which they 'fire'. This enables the representation of *cat* to be selected. It also ensures that the phonological representation of *cat* receives the most activation and so on down through the system.

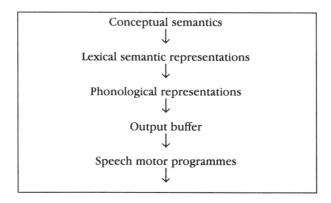

Figure 2.1.1 A model of single word production.

Of course, many processing questions remain unanswered by this model, such as:

- How does each box, or component, accomplish its task?
- What is the processing sequence of events?
- Is semantic information processed entirely before phonology or do the two interact?

We might also ask how deficits to the different components of the system manifest and whether those manifestations vary in children and adults. While we cannot give definitive answers to any of these questions, we can gather some hints from people experiencing word finding difficulties.

The semantic problems displayed by people with brain damage give us some insight into how the semantic system sets about its task. We know that a number of these individuals can process certain types of information better than others. For example, some can produce the names of objects better than living things (see for example Sheridan and Humphreys 1993); while others show the inverse pattern (Sacchett and Humphreys 1992). These dissociations suggest that semantic information may be organised categorically, possibly according to how it was acquired (Allport 1985, Caramazza *et al.* 1990). Thus information about the appearance of objects, acquired through vision or visual description, may be represented in its own sector of the system. A deficit to this sector will particularly impair items which are largely defined by their appearance, which would be true for many animals and natural phenomena. This impairment, therefore, may give rise to the categorical effect described above, in that we would expect that living things will be poorly named, while objects, which are largely defined by function, will be relatively preserved.

The impoverished retrieval of certain types of semantic information might also explain some semantic errors. Consider an example in which an aphasic person is trying to name *swan*. Normally, visual semantic information, such as *white* and *long neck*, will become available, together with categorical information, such as *bird* and behavioural information such as *flies*, *swims*, etc. Supposing there is a deficit in the retrieval of visual information. This would create a situation in which any bird which lives on water could be named. In other words, the person is just as likely to say *duck* as *swan*, indeed more so given its higher frequency.

Semantic errors also occur in child language disorder. However, the origins of such errors may differ. In the case of adults, semantic representations have been fully established, although the deficit has now impaired those representations or blocked access to them. This may not be the case for children. Here, the deficit may prevent normal representations from being formed. In other words, the child's representation for *swan* may be underspecified or contain idiosyncratic features. If this were the case, we would expect some consistency in the child's errors; i.e. *swan* will always be misnamed or misunderstood and the same types of semantic errors will occur from one occasion to the next.

Another question concerns the time course of processing, and specifically whether semantic and phonological processing occur in sequence or concurrently. Word finding errors are again informative here. When we analyse the semantic errors produced by unimpaired speakers we find that many are also related phonologically to the target, and more so than would be expected by chance (Dell 1988). This evidence suggests that we have to modify our model to permit some kind of interaction or feedback between the levels. We might illustrate this via an example in which a person is trying to name a pencil. Normally a range of features at the semantic level are activated. These, in turn, relay activation to all words in the lexicon which share those features. Thus *crayon*, *paint*, and *pen* all receive some activation. In the normal course of events, *pencil*, as the target, will receive the most activation and will 'fire'. However, imagine that the semantic information is in some way reduced or degraded so that none of the words, including the target, receives enough activation to be selected. Instead, a number of candidates are partially activated and these, in turn, partially activate segments of their phonology. Now an error is likely. Suppose the model allows some feedback between the levels. Thus the segments of phonology feed activation back to the possible words. Two of the candidates share phonological segments, namely *pen* and *pencil*. As a result, they receive the most feedback activation. This may be enough to fire the target. However, if it is not, *pen* is clearly the most likely error.

It seems that our basic model needs considerable elaboration, partly to illuminate what happens at each level and partly to allow for more complex and bidirectional communication between the levels. This has implications for how we apply the model when investigating and treating word finding problems. For example, the sequential model predicts that word finding could break down because of a problem at one level of the system, or in one of the connections between levels. We would expect these different deficits to manifest in relatively distinct ways. For example, people with a semantic deficit should reveal semantic errors (which should also occur on input), while those with a pure phonological deficit should reveal semantic strengths and a tendency to make phonological errors.

If we accept the more interactive model we cannot expect deficits to be quite so pure. Now we have to entertain the possibility that a deficit at one level of processing may have significant consequences for another. For example, an inability to access phonology will deprive the semantic level of feedback activation, which could result in the premature fading of semantic information. This might be particularly true in cases of child language disorder, where the deficit occurs in the context of a developing system. Thus, for example, a phonological deficit may inhibit the development of normal semantic representations, precisely because the semantic features are prevented from relaying their activation to a consistent phonological destination. Put differently, the semantic features of *swan* cluster together partly because they converge on one phonological representation. Without that representation, the clustering may be compromised.

The implications for therapy are also different. Even if we can pin down the deficit to one relatively distinct level of processing, we cannot be sure that targeting therapy at that level is necessarily the right thing to do. It may be more appropriate to exploit the better preserved areas of the system. This might be achieved through multi-dimensioned therapy tasks. For example, the person may be asked to judge the meaning of the word and access information about its phonology or its orthography. Such tasks presumably exploit the multiple connections within the system and thereby give the person the best opportunity for tapping into whatever strengths they have. Interestingly, this approach was adopted in both the studies that follow.

Chapter 2.2
When is a rolling pin a 'roll the pen': a clinical insight into lexical problems

SADIE LEWIS AND JANE SPEAKE

In 1993, Chiat and Hunt presented a study of a child with word finding problems, phonological errors and occasional semantic errors. A close psycholinguistic analysis of his language system generated evidence of impairments at several processing stages. Rather than hypothesising multiple deficits, Chiat and Hunt argued that the connections between processing levels were impaired. However, even with this hypothesis, it was not clear how to remediate the difficulties:

> Psycholinguistic investigation does not have direct implications for effective intervention, even if we can identify the source of impairment in processing, this does not determine whether and how that impairment can be remediated. (Chiat and Hunt 1993)

Clearly further investigations are needed to explore the links between a psycholinguisitc 'diagnosis' and the actual content of treatment.

Despite this caution, the work of Chiat and Hunt encouraged a number of clinicians to attempt therapy focusing on the links between processing levels. This was especially true for the link between the phonological and semantic lexical storage systems: **semantic–phonological therapy**. Activities aimed to link the semantics and phonology of a target word in an overt way. For example, clues games were used, where semantic and phonological information was given about a word for the child to guess what it was. This was thought to strengthen the word finding abilities of the child with access and storage difficulties. However, the efficacy of such therapy, and whether it taps into the right level of the child's processing system remain unexplored.

In the current study, two children with severe language disorders were investigated. Semantic and phonological assessments were carried out and therapy programmes devised. The aim was to provide some clinical insight into semantic–phonological therapy with these two children.

A second reason for undertaking these case descriptions was to investigate two children whose presenting symptomatology was similar.

Both children had severe word finding difficulties, with semantic and phonological errors and delayed word recall. Although the studies were carried out by two different therapists, the assessment framework was similar. This enabled us to hypothesise about whether the childrens' presenting symptomatology originated from the same processing deficit.

Case study 1: Richard

Richard was 8 years old at the start of the study. All developmental milestones were within normal limits with the exception of language development. He was referred for a language assessment at age 2 years 6 months. At this stage he used some nouns and relied on non-verbal cues to support comprehension. When he was 5 he was seen by an educational psychologist who confirmed the diagnosis of severe language disorder. When he was 6, he was recorded (statemented) and started to attend an extended learning support unit where additional support is given to the children within a mainstream school.

Richard is the younger of two children. He has an older sister who is doing well at school. His father works at a naval base and his mother works part time in an office. He comes from a very supportive home environment and there is no history of speech and language disorder in the family. All members of the family have a soft Scottish accent.

Previous therapy had adopted a 'developmental' and 'hole plug' approach. Richard's language was encouraged to move through a developmental pattern and delayed skills were specifically targeted in treatment. Work included concept development (e.g. *short/long*, *more/less*), comparatives (e.g. *big/small*), prepositions, tenses and auditory short term memory.

Initial observations and testing

Richard had clear articulation and good pragmatic skills. He was a popular member of his class and mixed well in the mainstream classroom. However, significant non-teaching adult support was needed for him to access the modified curriculum.

Richard was experiencing particular literacy problems. He was unable to develop alphabetic skills, which convert written letters into sounds. As a result he relied upon visual attack strategies, whereby he attempted to recognise whole word forms.

An overview of Richard's language abilities at 7 years 11 months was obtained by administering the Clinical Evaluation of Language Fundamentals – Revised (CELF-R). This comprises a number of receptive and expressive sub-tests which explore different levels of syntax, semantics and memory. His performance is summarised in Table 2.2.1. The CELF-R showed that Richard's receptive language was slightly stronger than his expressive skills. Observation suggested that his output suffered from severe word finding problems and limited sentence length and complexity. In contrast, he was able to support his input processing by exploiting visual cues and context.

Table 2.2.1 Pre-therapy results on the CELF-R (On all subtests the average range of the standard scores (SS) is 7–13 and the percentile rank (PR) is 16–84. For the composite scores, the average range standard score is 85–115; the average percentile rank is 16–84)

Receptive subtests
1. Linguistic concepts
Task: The child must interpret and carry out instructions which require processing of specific linguistic concepts, such as 'either … or', 'if … then'.
SS   5
PR   5

2. Sentence structure
Task: The child listens to sentences of increasing complexity and must identify the correct picture from a choice of four. Different structures are assessed,such as negatives and passives.
SS   5
PR   9

3. Oral directions
Task: The child must interpret, recall and carry out oral commands of increasing length and complexity, for example, 'Point to the small circle on the right of the black triangle'.
SS   5
PR   5

Expressive subtests
1. Formulated sentences
Task: The child must formulate a sentence around one or two given words. A picture is also presented as a prompt.
SS   3
PR   1

2. Recalling sentences
Task: The child must repeat sentences of increasing length and complexity, for example 'The dog chased the ball, and the cat didn't follow'.
SS   3
PR   1

3. Word structure
Task: This subtest looks at a child's knowledge and use of morphological rules and forms. It involves sentence completion e.g. 'This woman teaches. She is called a …'
SS   3
PR   1

Composite scores

	SS	PR
Receptive score	67	1
Expressive score	50	1
Total score	56	1

Age equivalent < 5 years

Investigations of the production deficit

Informal observation and the CELF suggested that Richard's communication problems stemmed mainly from his production deficit. To gain
more insight into the quality of Richard's output a picture description
sample was collected and analysed (see Table 2.2.2).

Table 2.2.2 Sample of Richard's expressive language in a picture description task
(Key: R = Richard; T = Therapist; - = approximately ½ second)

Making gingerbread men

R: The - - - it's a spoon - mixing it - - and there's a knife, a/sp/a fork - a egg -
sugar and salt - and the roll the salt and the roll, roll the pen - the pen to
roll the thing out - and - - and the - - - and the - - um

T: This one? (indicating second picture) Or have you not finished that one?
(indicating second picture)

R: Not finished that one

T: OK, Which bit are you stuck with? (R points to part of picture) Like a
shape, a cutter

R: Cutter. And the cutter - - - the - - thing - - and it's cooked - it's cooked - -
and it's hot.

T: It is hot

R: And it's got little um - - little hot, hot things

T: What's going to happen next? What's going to happen to the gingerbread
men?

R: Eat them

Making a cup of coffee

R: The lady - - the man pouring - um - - - tea - in the cup - and the - jug - -and
the jug - - water goes and the hot water goes in the jug and you press it
and you pour it and you drink it

Cat stalking a fish

R: Door is open - and the fish is in the gold fish - - and the cat's looked at
the fish and the cat - um - trying to get

T: What has Mrs Lewis done? (Pictures have been placed in the wrong order)
Try that

R: Messed up! The cat is looked at the fish and the cat seed the fish and the
gold fish is broken - it's knocked down

T: And, what do you see walking back?

R: Cat's foot prints

T: Cat's foot prints, that is right. What do you think happened to the fish?

R: Dead

T: Well, what do cats do with fish?

R: Swallow them - eat them

T: Eat them. Do you think the cat ate the fish?

R: Don't know

Richard's output displayed the following lexical difficulties:

- semantic errors, such as '*jug*' for *kettle*
- phonological errors, such as '*roll the pen*' for *rolling pin*
- delayed recall, repetitions and hesitations
- non-specific language – *it/that/thing, put/get/do*
- perseverations.

In addition, Richard had a very limited vocabulary and clearly did not know some words (e.g. goldfish bowl). This was confirmed by the British Picture Vocabulary Scales (BPVS). This test of receptive vocabulary showed a 2 year delay.

To identify the level of breakdown causing Richard's lexical problems several informal tests were administered. Owing to the large proportion of in-class semantic errors, his semantic system was hypothesised to be a level of difficulty and therefore investigated. Similarly, his phonological errors and literacy problems indicated that there may be covert phonological problems. This hypothesis was also followed up in assessment.

Assessments of semantic processing

Yes/no judgement

Richard was shown a picture of either an object or an action which the therapists named. Half the offered nouns or verbs were correct and half incorrect. For example, the picture might show a brush and the therapist would say 'comb'. Wherever close semantic distractors were presented he accepted them as correct names for the pictures.

Category generation

Richard was asked to name items within a given category. He found this extremely difficult and could rarely produce more than two or three items with frequent perseverations (e.g. clothes: '*jeans ..., shirt ..., T-shirt ..., vest ..., vest ..., granddad's shirt ..., no more*').

Semantic links assessment (Lewis 1994)

In this task Richard was shown an array of five pictures and had to identify which picture round the outside went best with the one in the middle (see Figure 2.2.1). He was also asked to give as many reasons as he could for the association. Out of 28 items, Richard correctly identified 21 associations, which was close to the average performance achieved by 7 year old controls on the same task (Lewis 1994). However, Richard did differ from the controls in his explanations. Children with no language problems gave an average of 84 explanations for their associations, whereas Richard could only give 12. Furthermore, many of his explanations were non-specific (e.g. 'they go together because they are the same').

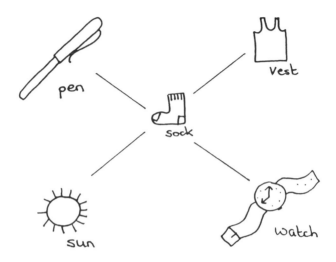

Figure 2.2.1 Semantic links assessment.

Conclusions from the semantic assessments

Richard's performance on the semantic links assessment demonstrated that he had some non-verbal semantic knowledge as he was able to associate items. However, his ability to give explanations was very limited. This could be due either to underspecified semantic associations or an inability to express them. Similarly, Richard's poor performance on the category naming task might reflect reduced semantic knowledge or an inability to map accessed semantic information on to phonological forms.

If Richard's semantic information was reduced we would expect problems even on pure input tasks. This was indeed the case, since he made several errors on the yes/no judgement task in which he had to distinguish between semantically related words. We therefore hypothesised that Richard had a semantic deficit. This might take the form of undifferentiated semantic information, giving rise to 'fuzzy' semantic representations, and/or might be a problem of access, in which Richard's capacity to retrieve semantic information was reduced.

Assessments of phonological processing

A range of phonological processing tasks were administered to assess Richard's input skills, the status of his internal phonological representations and his ability to realise those representations in different output tasks.

Minimal pair task (Bridgeman and Snowling 1988)

Richard was asked to listen to two words and say if they were the same or different. Both real and matched non-words were used, so a comparison could be made between his ability to analyse familiar and new phonological material (see Table 2.2.3).

Richard was well above chance with the real words. In contrast, he showed severe problems analysing new phonological material (i.e. non-words). This suggested that he was using lexical knowledge to support auditory processing. With non-words, no such knowledge was available, i.e. he had no internal representation which could help him to analyse or retain the two word forms. As a result, his judgements were at chance. Richard's processing of words and non-words was investigated further through a repetition task.

Table 2.2.3 Minimal pair task

Segment discrimination (final phoneme varied)	
Real words (e.g. *loss/lot, wet/wet*)	12/15
Non-words (e.g. *voss/vot, woos/woos*)	7/15
Sequence discrimination (sequence of final two phonemes varied)	
Real words (e.g. *lost/lots, west/west*)	12/15
Non-words (e.g. *vost/vots, woots/woots*)	8/15

Non-word and real word repetition

Richard was asked to repeat 10 words and 10 non-words which were 'matched' for phonological complexity. The non-words and words were given on separate occasions to avoid priming. Richard had severe difficulty imitating the non-words. However, he could easily imitate the real words. Table 2.2.4 shows his responses. There were no output constraints at a low level inhibiting the pronunciation of the non-words, as the real words with similar phonological sequences were imitated accurately. Therefore, poor analysis of phonological material on input was hypothesised to be the cause. With the real words the input component of the task was supported by his own internal representations, hence the better performance.

Initial sound detection

Richard was presented with three pictures and asked which ones start with the same sound. In order to carry out this task, he had to recognise each picture and access the word's phonological representation. He then had to segment the initial sound and compare it to the other pictures. He scored 14/20, which was well above chance. This showed that he had some segmentation skills and was able to carry out the basic manipulations required. However, this was not consistent and errors were made.

Table 2.2.4 Real word/non-word repetition task

Non-word	Imitation	Real word	Imitation
vɛəə	vɛfə	Feather	✓
glɒgətɪjəl	'crocodile'	Crocodile	✓
lɛwɪgɒbdə	lɛvɜ	Helicopter	✓
dɛwəvəʊd	dɛvɜ	Telephone	✓
kleɪfi	'crocodile'	Gravy	✓
əgrɛəwijəb	ægʌd	Aquarium*	ækrɪəm
gæləd	'cracker'	Carrot	✓
ʌŋgiɛwə	əŋgɑʊɜ	Umbrella	✓
tʃəleɪdiəb	'chair'	Geranium*	dʒɛrʌm
bɔgjubaɪd	'football'	Porcupine	'pocket'

* a non-word for Richard.

Rhyme detection

Richard was presented with five pictures, one in the middle of the page and four surrounding it. He was asked which of the surrounding pictures rhymed with the one in the middle. The four options consisted of the target rhyme, a phonological distracter (initial sound link), a semantic distractor and an unrelated distracter. Richard identified 5/14 rhymes. His errors were mostly semantic (7/14) with two phonological ones. Seven year olds with normal language development found an average of 12 rhymes, with their errors being primarily phonological (Lewis 1994). Thus Richard, at the age of 8, performed worse than these younger control subjects and with a different error pattern.

Richard demonstrated that he had a very underdeveloped awareness of rhyme. His links were mostly semantic and the idea of linking words according to their phonological make up seemed to be minimal. This was further confirmed by the next task.

Rhyme generation

Richard was asked to think of as many words as he could that rhymed with a given word. Some of his attempts are given in Table 2.2.5. Despite his achievement with the first word, it is clear that rhyme links were not established. Instead he often gave a semantic association. Richard's poor appreciation of rhyme suggested that any phonological component of therapy should target the easier link of 'initial sound', rather than rhyme.

Conclusions from phonological assessments

Richard had an interesting range of strengths and weaknesses in phonological processing. The phonological assessments showed that there were input difficulties at the level of auditory analysis as he had difficulty discriminating and repeating non-words. However, he was able to use lexical/semantic information to overcome some of these problems, which led to a superior performance on the same tests with real words. On the output side, it was difficult for him to access his internal phonological representations and compare them, as shown with the poor initial phoneme and rhyme detection. Again, it seems that he tries to use information from elsewhere in his system to overcome difficulties. For example, in the rhyme generation task he triggers production by using semantic associations (*bin* → 'basket', *key* → 'door').

Table 2.2.5 Attempted rhyme generation

Given word	Richard's response
Hat	*mat, pat, rat, fat, dat*
Key	*cat, pat, door, draw, more*
Comb	*coat, mat, pat*
Bin	*basket*
Shell	*crab, rap, sell, rab*
Draw	*braw, door, raw*
Log	*draw, braw, bit someone*
Sew	*sewing*

Semantic–phonological integration

The tests so far indicated that Richard could use semantic cues to generate output. Thus he had some, albeit limited, success on the category generation task and used semantic links inappropriately in the rhyme task above. He could also draw upon phonological associations, in that some rhyming words were produced. However, these skills were very inconsistent and limited.

We were interested in whether Richard's output would improve if he was given cues containing both semantic and phonological information, i.e 'What is in the sky and starts with /m/'. In fact, as the following examples show, Richard could only act upon one element of the cue:

T: What is in the sky and starts with /m/?
R: Sun
T: What starts with /s/ and you use to cut wood?
R: Saucer

He could use both semantic and phonological information individually to aid naming, but could not integrate the two types of information to generate a target.

Overall assessment conclusions

Richard displayed problems at several processing levels. There was an 'early' deficit in auditory analysis. This deficit was less significant for real words, presumably because Richard could call upon stored lexical/semantic information to assist processing. However, there was evidence that some of this information was itself impaired. Richard made errors on all semantic tasks, suggesting that he had underdeveloped or unorganised semantic representations. His ability to access stored phonological representations was also poor, as was seen in the initial sound and rhyme detection tasks. The final cueing task showed that it was very difficult for Richard to integrate semantic and phonological information in output. We concluded that not only was semantic and phonological information impaired, but also the links between these systems.

Therapy hypothesis

In order for Richard to access lexical items more easily and accurately, their representations must be more defined. He had unorganised semantic information about many items and this provided insufficient semantic drive to access the correct phonological representation. In addition, his phonological representations may be fuzzy due to his input processing problems. Therefore, it was hypothesised that therapy should aim to improve the structure of the semantic lexicon and strengthen phonological representations. In addition, the link between the semantic and phonological representations would be overtly worked at to try to ensure that when he knew what he wanted to say (semantic knowledge) he could map this on to the correct phonological form in his phonological lexicon (**semantic–phonological therapy**).

Therapy

Owing to clinical time pressures it was only possible to see Richard for one individual and two group sessions a week. This took place in school with follow-up materials given for home and class work. Therapy lasted for one year, term time only.

Aim 1: To develop semantic knowledge (group work)

- **Associating vocabulary** Richard was shown an array of pictures and had to find two pictures that went together and generate three more associated items. For example, 'give me three more – socks, shoes ...'
- **Linking** A set of object cards were turned over one at a time. Richard had to name the object and then say what you do with it (e.g. 'orange – eat it', 'sock – wear it'). If he was correct he could keep the card. It was then another child's turn to take and name a card. In the next group the same set of cards were used and their location given (e.g. 'mug – kitchen', 'flower – garden'). Other links subsequently

explored were category (e.g. 'dress – clothes', 'apple – food'), attribute (e.g. 'soup – hot', 'pencil – long') and part (e.g. 'lorry – wheels', 'shoe – laces'). In this way a range of semantic information was built up around each lexical item.

- **Explanation of links – why things go together** Richard was shown several pictures that could be linked to a central item (**semantic links**, Bigland and Speake 1992). He was asked to identify the associated items and explain why they went together, e.g. 'shoes + socks – because you wear them, they go on your feet'. This built on the knowledge gained in the linking game described above and basic explanations were soon given.
- **Picture sorting** Richard was given several pictures to sort according to given criteria (**semantic connections**, Speake and Bigland-Lewis 1995). For example, animals/not animals, animals/clothes, pets/not pets, wild/not wild, farm/not farm, pets/wild/farm. If needed, preparatory work was done through stories and discussing personal experiences (e.g. school trip to a farm).
- **Odd one out** Three pictures were shown to Richard and he had to find and explain why one was the odd one out (**semantic connections**, Speake and Bigland-Lewis 1995). Initially one item was out of category. This was slowly graded to within-category judgements. For example: dog, mouse, sock; lion, cat, elephant
- **Composite pictures** Richard was shown composite pictures around a theme (**talking semantics**, Lewis and Bird 1995). He had to identify which items were linked with the theme and explain why. Themes included cold, heavy, handles, open/closed.
- **Opposites** This was played as a quiz. The children had to give the opposite to a provided word and draw it when possible. For example: Therapist: long; Richard: short (drew short hair)

These activities were all done in a group. There were three children, each with very different abilities. However, they offered mutual support and respected one another's contributions. They listened to one another's explanations of links and commented on how appropriate they were. Therefore, even when it was not Richard's turn he was actively involved in semantic reasoning.

Aim 2: To develop phonological processing skills

This component of therapy aimed to improve Richard's analysis of phonological sequences, and improve his skills in accessing phonological representations. We also aimed to give him some ability to reflect upon the phonological structure of words in a conscious way. Initial sounds were focused on, using the 'Letterland' materials (Stephanie 1993). Each week a single phoneme was worked on and the following activities were carried out around it. Again treatment took place in groups.

- A **Letterland character story** was read. The words starting with the week's sound were emphasised.
- The children looked at the picture accompanying the story and took it in turns to find something that started with the sound.
- **Yes/no judgement** The therapist said a word and Richard had to judge if it started with the target sound. Close phonological distractors were used, e.g. P – 'pig, book, black, pocket, pillow'.
- Sorting pictures according to their **initial sound**. This was a silent game and required the children to reflect on their stored phonological representation.
- Generating by **initial sound**. Richard had to recall and then draw something starting with the target sound. When problems arose semantic clues were given. If he still found it difficult, the character's picture was referred to (see above) and Richard could find something to copy.
- Identification of which items on a composite picture start with a given sound (**talking phonology**, Lewis and Papier 1996). Both semantic and phonological (rhyme) distractors were contained in the picture. Richard was encouraged to focus on the sound at the start of the word.
- **Cued articulation** (see page 33) was introduced. However, Richard showed reluctance to use this and it was not continued.

Aim 3: To develop semantic–phonological mapping (individual therapy)

- These tasks integrated semantic and phonological work, i.e. semantic activities were done around the Letterland characters and the semantic group work was revised now with the addition of initial sound work. For example, during the opposites topic, the pictures were revised and the initial sound was requested, and during the Letterland /p/ week, the pictures were revised and their function, location, category, attributes and parts were named.
- Clues games were carried out. For example, 'Think of something at the seaside that starts with s'. Turn taking was encouraged.

Outcomes

Richard enjoyed all therapy sessions. He found the semantic group most challenging, as both the other children had stronger skills. However, this did not detract from his motivation. He regularly asked which Letterland characters we would be reading about that week and he was known to do some preparation work for the session (e.g. asking his teacher if his name had the sound in it). All activities were presented within his ability and cues given when needed. Initially semantic information was added, then additional phonological information (e.g. syllable structure). If he continued to have problems a picture was found to help him remember the word. If this was not possible, options were given, e.g. 'is it hot or cold?'

After a year, the sequencing cards were looked at again to help evaluate change (see Table 2.2.6). The changes noted were as follows:

Table 2.2.6 Sample of Richard's expressive language following one year of therapy

Making gingerbread men
R: The spoon is in the bowl - mixing up with sugar and rolling up - rolling pin - and put it in the - - in the - - um
T: What do you do with this thing Richard?
R: Cook. Cooked.
T: Cook
R: The cookery
T: A cooker
R: And the gingerbread is made
T: What is going to happen next?
T: You eat them

Making a cup of coffee
R: Into the cup - and the taps on and pour the kettle in the cup - in the - - tap and - switch the kettle on and then you pour then the cup is drinking

Cat stalking a fish
R: The s - the s - the door is open the fish is in the pond. The cat's coming out, in then the fish - the cat's seen the fish, the cat walked to the fish and jumped on the table to see the fish - the cat put the paw in the water and the cat ran away and eat the fish
T: Do you think he's eaten the fish?
R: Yep
T: I think he has hasn't he. What's happened to the bit down there?
R: Broked
T: Do you know what it is?
R: No
T: Pond, fish bowl or tank?
R: Fish bowl
T: Fish bowl, well done

Cutting a tree down
R: The tree is up and the re ... the - man sawed the tree down - - the tree's broked down - and the man put another tree on
T: He is isn't he. Planting another tree - and this tree is?
R: Fall down
T: Fall down

Playing football on the pavement
R: The boy is kicking the ball on the pavement. The ball bounced on the road and the ball - - the boy watched the ball and the - - boy with the - man seed - the - ur - - ball - the two man - they boy and the man looked and listened and looked and you get the ball

- There were fewer semantic and phonological errors. Words which had caused problems during the first administration, such as *rolling pin* and *gingerbread men*, were now achieved. He was more cueable and could select target words from given alternatives.
- The rate of word finding improved and there was much less hesitation and repetition, e.g. in 'Making coffee' there were 7 hesitations initially, compared with 4 at follow up.

Other changes were noted through more general observation, and through a detailed discussion with his mother:

- He was more fluent and commented that the words don't get stuck so often.
- He had more communicative confidence and was observed to be a more active member of discussion both in the classroom and playground. He attempted sentences in front of the whole class. Initially he was reluctant to do this and preferred a small group, but during the year change was noted.
- His basic alphabetic/phonic skills were improving and this was aiding literacy development. He was able to sound out the word and use this in conjunction with the semantic knowledge gained from the picture and story to help work out what the word was.

Richard continued to have significant word finding difficulties. However, when experiencing these problems, he was now able to provide semantic and some phonological information when questioned. There was some evidence that this was the beginning of a self-cue strategy:

    T: What do you do with it?
    R: My rabbit will live in it
    T: Where do you find it?
    R: In the garden
    T: Is it a short or a long word?
    R: Short
    T: Does it start with /h/ or /w/?
    R: h – I think... yes hutch... Wolf Man [rabbit's name] will live in a hutch

Following years of speech and language therapy, many people believed that Richard's language had reached a plateau. However, using semantic–phonological therapy good improvements seemed to be made.

Case study 2: Rosie

Rosie was 7 years old at the start of the study (and just 8 when the therapy took place). She was born at full term but had a low birth weight (2.4 kg) and her mother was diabetic during pregnancy. Rosie was born with a congenital deformity of the right foot (talipes equinovarus). This was corrected with a splint, strapping and surgery. She is one of two children and has a baby sister. Her father works in a restaurant and her mother is at home. Cantonese is the first language spoken at home. Her father speaks very little English but her mother is fluent. There is some support from the extended family.

Rosie was a healthy child but had a history of ear infections which affected her hearing. She was first referred for ear, nose and throat (ENT) examinations in June 1993 and in July had her tonsils and adenoids removed. Examination showed significant middle ear damage resulting from previous infections and she was fitted with a hearing aid in her left ear. She later had a grommet inserted into her right ear and subsequently was fitted with bilateral hearing aids. Rosie manages her hearing aids well and shows no difficulty at all in acuity.

Rosie was referred for speech and language therapy by the ENT department at the age of 5. The therapist reported that she had a severe language delay and took her on for regular blocks of therapy. Intervention included a school visit with an interpreter who confirmed that Rosie's Cantonese was as delayed as her English. She was using short, telegrammatic utterances with some word order problems evident in both languages. She had poor vocabulary and marked word finding problems. She also showed severe comprehension difficulties both in English and Cantonese.

At 6½ Rosie saw the educational psychologist who administered the Wechsler pre-school and primary scale of intelligence. Her verbal IQ was 71 (3rd centile) and her performance IQ was 88 (21st centile). This discrepancy was felt to be indicative of a specific language disorder. Rosie was referred to the language unit where she is currently placed.

Initial observations

Rosie had good attention, was cooperative and well motivated. She had frequent difficulties in understanding during conversation and in manipulating semantic information (e.g. clues games were very difficult for her). Also, her syntax was disordered with significant word order problems. Examples of expressive language:

> cos my baby was trying get run around with the walk chair
> (my baby was trying to run with the baby walker)
> when she was lucky she put on her flowers and trees as well
> (the lady next door had put Christmas lights in her garden)

A general picture of her language skills was derived by administering the CELF-R. Table 2.2.7 shows the results (see Table 2.2.1 for explanations of the subtests). This test confirmed that Rosie's production difficulties were more severe than her receptive difficulties. These were therefore focused on in the detailed investigations which followed.

Table 2.2.7 Rosie's results on the CELF-R at 7 years (On all subtests the average standard score (SS) range is 7–13; the average percentile rank (PR) range is 16–84. For composite scores, the average SS is 85–115, the average PR is 16–84)

	SS	PR
Receptive subtests		
Linguistic concepts	3	1
Sentence structure	6	9
Oral directions	9	37
Expressive subtests		
Formulated sentences	3	1
Recalling sentences	3	1
Word structure	4	2
Composite scores		
Receptive language	74	4
Expressive language	50	1
Total average score	63	1

Investigations of production

Rosie's articulation was normal and she had no history of peripheral speech production problems. However, she had severe word finding problems showing delayed recall, in-class semantic and phonological errors. Her production also seemed hampered by conceptual and planning problems, particularly when she attempted story telling (see Table 2.2.8).

Table 2.2.8 Examples of Rosie's story telling. Excerpt from 'Goldilocks and the three bears' – telling the story with no picture support Key: R = Rosie; T = Therapist

R: Once upon a time there was three bears ... and three bears
T: Who were the bears?
R: Mummy's bear and daddy bear and the baby bear ...
T: Can you remember what they did?
R: No, in the first picture ... I don't know
T: I think that mummy bear made something for breakfast – Can you remember?
R: Yes – bake it for breakfast then, they go to bed, when they finished their ...
T: Did they go to bed or out for a walk?
R: No – not in the first pictures

Rosie's production difficulties were explored further via two standardised tests: the Renfrew Action Picture Test and the Renfrew Word Finding Vocabulary Scale. In the first, Rosie was required to answer a number of questions about 10 action pictures. This test revealed immaturities of both syntax and lexical retrieval. Her information score was between 6 and 12 months delayed and her grammar score was over 2 years delayed. The second test was a simple picture naming task. One this, Rosie's score was even more delayed (at chronological age 7 years 5 months her age equivalent was 4;6). Her responses included both phonological and semantic errors (eg /geɪ/ and /keɪ/ for *kite* and '*goat*' for *cow*). There were also several words, such as *scarecrow*, which she did not know.

Rosie's poor word finding extended to verbs. In an informal task Rosie was shown 48 action pictures and asked to say what was happening. She labelled 38 accurately, although with some items she showed delayed recall. Errors included underspecification (eg '*doing*' for *lighting candles*), semantic ('*baking*' for *mixing*) and phonological (/struɪŋ/ for *stroking the dog*).

The production tests so far suggested that Rosie's lexical problems were a major contributor to her communication problems. There was already evidence of difficulties at both the semantic and phonological levels. The semantic evidence included the presence of semantic errors and her poor comprehension. The phonological evidence was more contradictory. On one side she made frequent phonological errors (see Table 2.2.9). On the other side was the evidence of her reading. Although Rosie's reading comprehension was poor, her accuracy was age appropriate and she could read aloud fluently. It seemed that she was reading largely without meaning, by using good phonological decoding skills. It seemed that a more detailed investigation of both her semantic and phonological skills was warranted.

Table 2.2.9 Examples of Rosie's phonological errors

Target	Production	Target	Production
Tower	'tɔl ɔl	Slippers	'slɪ pɪ s t
Jelly	'tʃɛri	Yacht	jɒtʃ
Dog	'dɒk	Railings	'sleɪlɪd
Clown	'klaʊd	Kite	geɪ keɪt
Drawer	'drɔl	Tractor/bus	trʌst
Sparrow	'slaʊwaʊ	Towel	taʊwə
Badge	baedʒəz	Roller-skate	'raʊlə skaʊt
Barclay's Bank	'bɜ d eɪ bank	Corn	'kɒn
Knitting	'nitɪŋ	Stroking	'struɪŋ
Ironing	ʌ'juɪŋ	Web	'wɛp
Nails	'sneɪlz	Walker's cheese and onion crisps	*cheese of* /krɪbz/ *in a* /weɪkəz/

Assessments of semantic processing

Lexical comprehension tests

If there was a central semantic impairment, we would anticipate lexical comprehension difficulties. This was probed for in two receptive tests. In the British Picture Vocabulary Scale Rosie was required to point to one of four pictures in response to a spoken word. At 8 years, Rosie's age equivalent score on this test was 4;6. In addition to poor comprehension, this score indicated that her vocabulary acquisition was very delayed, possibly because of her hearing impairment and bilingualism as well as her specific language disorder.

In the second test Rosie was shown verb pictures which the therapist named, either correctly or with a semantic error. Rosie had to judge whether or not the correct verb label had been given. She made 4 errors in 60 items (accepting *knit* for *sew*, *ride* for *drive*, *push* for *pull* and *catch* for *throw*). She self-corrected on two items *drink/eat*, *walk/run*.

Semantic links assessment (see Case study 1 for details)

Rosie identified 24 out of the 28 target associations, which was appropriate for her age. However, whereas the control 7 year olds gave an average of 84 correct explanations, Rosie gave only 42. Most of her explanations were based on the function of items, e.g. *balloon* goes with *kite* 'because they are things you can play when its wind blow'.

Category generation

Rosie's ability to generate items in a given semantic category was extremely limited e.g. she could only think of five animals in one minute.

Conclusions from semantic assessments

Rosie's performance on semantic tasks was broadly similar to Richard's. She fell into semantic traps (i.e. was confused by words with closely associated meanings) which supported the view that her semantic system was underspecified. In addition to semantic confusion it became evident during assessment that there were words which Rosie had never learnt at all (either in English or Cantonese). This was supported by discussion with her mother. Rosie seemed to have limited knowledge about known words as shown by her performance on the semantic links task. She seems to have rather stereotyped associations based around the function of items.

Assessments of phonological processing

Given Rosie's skills in decoding phonology when reading it was evident that she had some strengths in this area. This was confirmed during assessment.

Minimal pair judgement task (Bridgeman and Snowling 1988)

Rosie scored 60/60, indicating no difficulty in discriminating real or non-words in this same–different judgement task.

Non-word repetition

Rosie managed well with single syllable words including clusters. Multisyllable words were more difficult but there were only a few errors.

Initial sound detection

Rosie was able to match and sort pictures by initial sounds and made no errors in the task.

Rhyme detection

Rosie was shown an array of five pictures, one in the centre of the page and four round it. She was asked which of the four surrounding pictures rhymed with the central one. She scored 10 out of 14 correct which is within the average range for a child of her age (Lewis 1994). Two of her errors were alliterative, i.e. the words shared first sounds, and two involved the selection of a semantically related item.

Rhyme generation

Rosie's results were variable. For example, for *cat* she produced '*pat, bat, rat, tat, drat, wat, mat, sat*' but for *wall* she kept losing the word and after several false starts was not able to think of any rhymes. The difficulty may have been in holding on to the target word rather than inherently to do with rhyme.

Conclusions from the phonological assessments

Rosie's performance on the tests of phonological processing indicated competence in a range of tasks. She could discriminate related phonological sequences on input, and reproduce them in repetition. She could also access phonological representations and analyse them for initial sound and rhyme. Her strong performance does not preclude the possibility of earlier difficulties, which are now resolved.

Overall assessment conclusions and therapy hypothesis

Rosie had semantic problems affecting comprehension and word finding. The phonological aspect of Rosie's difficulty was also investigated. As with Richard, Rosie had never had any articulation difficulties. Assessment showed that her phonological processing skills were generally intact. However, Rosie did produce phonological errors, which in adults would be classed as literal paraphasias. We hypothesised that the semantic drive was too weak to access the full phonology of the word. However, the mechanism leading to this difficulty was still unclear. One possibility was that she simply did not know the word well enough. Another was that poor semantic organisation generated 'semantic noise' which obstructed access. If it is the first explanation, then simple over-learning of vocabulary should improve the naming and decrease the phonological errors. If the problem is more complex, then tasks aiming to increase semantic information and link that to phonological information might be more effective. This was explored in therapy.

Therapy

Therapy took place over 10 individual 30 minute sessions. Two sets of words were targeted using **semantic–phonological therapy** (SPT) and two sets using **familiarisation therapy** (FT). These were 'toys' and 'things with wheels', and 'furniture' and 'things with legs' respectively. Rosie's ability to name pictures of toys and furniture, and to generate items in the given categories of 'things with wheels' and 'things with legs' was assessed before and after therapy. Results are shown in tables 2.2.10–2.2.12.

Table 2.2.10 Semantic–phonological therapy: toys

Target	Production pre-therapy		Production post-therapy	
Ball	✓	A	✓	A
Balloon	✓	A	✓	A
Bricks	✓	A	✓	A
Computer	✓	A	✓	D
Penguin*	/pɪŋgwɪn/	PE	/pɪŋgwɪn/	PE
Doll	✓	A	✓	A
Pushchair	✓	A	✓	D
Doll's House	a house for a dolly✓	A	✓	A
Draughts	DK (game)	DK	/dras/	PE
Drum	✓	A	✓	A
Jack in the box	/jʌŋgl/ that makes you surprised	PE	✓	A
Puzzle	✓	A	✓	A
Kite	✓	A	✓	A
Puppet*	/mʌmɪt/	PE	✓	A
Roller skates**	sk - əeɪf - skeɪt rəuli - ʌəuli rəuk skeɪt - rəulɪŋ skeɪt	PE	✓	A
Skipping Rope	✓	A	✓	A
Soldier	/ʃəuldə/	PE	ʃəudʒə → ✓	C
Teddy	✓	A	✓	A
Toy truck	fire engine - car - caravan	S	✓	D
Yo-yo	✓	A	✓	A
Total named	**13**		**18**	

A, accurately named; PE, phonological error; C, self-corrected; U, underspecified; S, semantically related; PC, phonic cue given; D, delayed (slow) recall; DK, don't know.
* These may be mis-learnt rather than phonological errors because /pɪŋgwɪn/ and /mʌmɪt/ were used frequently when naming the items.
**Also produced as skating rolls, rolling skatings.

Table 2.2.11 Familiarisation therapy: furniture

Target	Production pre-therapy		Production post-therapy	
Armchair	chair - one person	U	✓	D
Bookshelf	✓	A	✓	A
Bunk beds	/bʌm/ bed	PE	/bʌmf/ beds *	PE
Bedside cabinet	desk - two desk	S	✓	A
Chair	✓	A	/stʃɛə/	PE
Coffee table	table (also D)	U	✓	A
Cot	✓	A	✓	D
Cupboard	✓	A	shelves - no - ✓	C
Desk	table – /dɛks/ – /dʌsk/	PE	✓	D
Double bed	bed	U	✓	A
Chest of drawers	wardrobe	S	let me think - DK - give me the 1st sound ⓟⓒ ✓	PC
Dresser	jam desk	S	✓	D
Dressing table	desk – drawers	S	dressing	U
Grandfather clock	clock	U	✓	A
Shelves	shelf ✓	A	✓	A
Single bed	big bed	U	✓	A
Sofa/settee	1) /tʃɛəʃ/ 2) ✓	C	✓	A
Stool	chair	S	1) /stʊʌl/ - no 2) ✓	C
Table	✓	A	✓	A
Wardrobe	✓	A	cupboard ... DK ... DK ... ⓟⓒ → ✓	PC
Total named	**8**		**15**	

* that one is my – my – kind of a what kind of bed ... [initial sound and syllable pattern given] ... – bed

Table 2.2.12 Item generation

Semantic–phonological therapy: things with wheels

Pre-therapy	Post-therapy
lorry	tractor
cars	bus
motorbike	car
bicycle	van
van	lorry
aeroplane	bicycle
	wheelchair
	pushchair
	motorbike
	bike
Total 6	**Total 10**

(contd)

Table 2.2.12 (contd)

Familiarisation therapy: things with legs

Pre therapy	Post-therapy
people	people
animals	grandad
pets	grandma
person	fox
children	monkey
	chair
	table
	settee
	armchair
Total 5	**Total 9**

The materials used in therapy consisted of picture category sets for 'toys' and 'furniture'; these were taken from Semantic Connections (Speake and Bigland-Lewis 1995), plus 'home made' games and the Usborne 1000 word book (Amery and Cartright 1989).

SPT for toys and things with wheels

The aim was to develop Rosie's semantic and phonological information about two sets of items and to integrate this information in order to improve her ability to name them.

1. Pictures were simply **named** and the syllable structure and initial sound of the word were discussed with Rosie. For example: 'here is a kite, it has one clap and starts with a "k". Rosie was encouraged to clap the words with the therapist, and to say the initial sound.
2. Pictures were **sorted** according to the number of syllables or initial sound. For example, three post boxes were put out labelled 1, 2 and 3. Rosie had to turn over a picture, clap the word and post it into the right box.
3. **Clues games** A set of pictures was put out and Rosie was given clues containing both phonological and semantic information. For example, 'it has three claps, starts with a "b" and has pedals'. She was encouraged to listen to all the information before finding the picture and guessing was discouraged. This was a turn-taking game and Rosie was also asked to give clues to the therapist. These clues had to contain both semantic and phonological information.
4. **Identification** of pictures from given sounds. Words were segmented into onset/rhyme or onset/nucleus/coda, and Rosie had to find the correct picture, e.g. b-all or b-a-ll.
5. **Pairs games** Two sets of identical pictures were placed face down on the table. In turns, Rosie and the therapist tried to find a pair, by

tuning over two cards. Every time a pair was found, the item was clapped, the initial (and later final) sound identified and some semantic features reinforced, e.g. 'van, it has one clap, it starts with "v" and it has 4 wheels. A postman might drive one.'

6. Identifying and matching **initial and final sounds**. Pictures were turned over, the initial or final sound identified and the correct grapheme found in a set of coloured plastic letters.

7. **Rhyming games** Using one and two syllable words, a picture was chosen and the word written clearly. Rosie was helped to generate words which rhymed with a target and these were also written. All rhymes generated were written but real words and non-words were clearly differentiated. For example, 'Teddy – ready, steady, heddy – that is a rhyme but it is not a real word'.

8. Identifying **vowels**, discriminating vowel sounds in words, and looking for similarities between words. Because the words were semantically rather than phonologically linked, possible work with vowels proved quite difficult to incorporate (because the phonology is so dissimilar). However, in two of the sessions Rosie was encouraged to think about the vowels. Words sharing vowels were pulled together by the therapist and Rosie was shown why they were similar.

9. Listening activity involving **yes/no judgement**. Prior to the therapy sessions covered in the study, Rosie had been very muddled when giving clues about 'wheels' and 'legs'. She was asked to listen to a list of items and identify whether or not they had wheels. If an item with wheels was correctly identified, it was clapped and sounded out.

FT for furniture and things with legs

This therapy aimed to train the names of two sets of items, to see whether this alone was enough to facilitate their production. The therapist attempted to ensure that additional phonological or semantic information was restricted as much as possible.

1. **Naming** Pictures of items were presented and named by the therapist and Rosie was encouraged to repeat the correct names. For 'things with legs' the therapist pointed out and named appropriate items. For example, 'here is a bed, it has legs, and so does a chair, there's a cat on the chair, she has legs too'.

2. **Identification of pictures** when named. Rosie's favourite game was the 'hiding game'. Pictures were 'hidden' around the room and she was asked to find specific items e.g. 'find the bunk beds'. Turn taking was included with Rosie giving instructions to the therapist which encouraged her production of the correct and specific name, for example, if Rosie said '*find the bed*', the therapist said 'which bed do you mean?'

3. **Lotto game**   This is a simple matching game: pictures are turned over and matched to a game board. Naming of items was encouraged and reinforced by the therapist.

4. **Identification/naming**   Using picture books (e.g. the Usborne 1000 word book Amery and Cartright 1989) and Rosie was asked to find and name all the things with legs on a page. Naming was reinforced, if necessary , by the therapist.

5. **'Stamper' game**   Using photocopied sets of pictures Rosie was asked to find particular items and mark them with a stamper pen, e.g. 'put a smiley face on the coffee table'.

6. **Fishing**   Pictures were attached to plastic fish and Rosie had to catch them with a magnetic rod and name the items she caught.

7. **Listening activity**   This involved yes/no judgements for items with legs. Rosie had to listen to a list and identify which items had legs.

Results of therapy

During therapy sessions Rosie was cooperative and well motivated. She had certain favourite games (for example, the 'hiding game' and using the stamper pens) but seemed to enjoy all activities. Having been at the language unit for nearly a year she was well used to individual and group therapy sessions.

The quantitative results of therapy are shown in tables 2.2.10–2.2.12. There were gains with both types of therapy. The numerical gain for the furniture (FT) names is greater. However, pre-therapy 5 of the furniture items were given underspecified labels, e.g. 'bed' for double, single and bunk beds, so the gain was in more detailed labelling. Gains in naming for toys (SPT) were reductions in the number of phonological errors and learning the words she did not know. These improvements would have more functional value since context usually aids comprehension of underspecified labels. It was interesting to note that during reassessment Rosie frequently asked *'what's the first sound?'* when stuck on a furniture (FT) item. It seemed that she was attempting to apply a strategy acquired in the SPT to these items. This in turn might suggest that the SPT had given Rosie skills which could potentially generalise beyond the specifically practised items.

Rosie's ability to generate items with wheels (SPT) and legs (FT) improved with both forms of therapy. Again, qualitative differences were evident between the two, and SPT resulted in more fluent and rapid naming.

Discussion

During initial observations, both children presented in a similar way. Both had severe word finding problems, which seemed as least partly underpinned by semantic problems. They also demonstrated phonological errors in the absence of any speech difficulties. However, upon closer examination, their profiles were quite different, particularly in terms of phonology. Richard revealed phonological processing difficulties at a number of levels and in both input and output tasks. In contrast, Rosie revealed a number of phonological skills. We therefore hypothesised that her phonological errors in output were largely the result of weak semantic drive. The therapy rationales were therefore different for each child despite original similarities.

For Richard, the rationale was to improve both semantic and phonological organisation and the mapping between the two levels. Rosie's therapy also incorporated considerable phonological work. However, we hypothesised that this encouraged her to draw upon a strength. In other words, good phonological skills were being used to improve semantic access again by explicitly associating a phonological form with semantic features of the word. Thus the therapy tasks used with the two children were often similar, although the rationales were different.

These case descriptions highlight the need for individual psycholinguistic profiles to be drawn up prior to therapy planning. This may not lead to radically new therapies, but does make the rationale for familiar treatments more explicit:

> We find ourselves using well-established therapy techniques but with new rationales (Chiat and Hunt 1993)

Both children showed some improvement following therapy, primarily in informal assessment and observation. Semantic–phonological therapy seemed to influence the ease and speed of word access. However, this was a clinical rather than experimental study and wider investigations of this type of therapy are needed to establish the validity of the approach and to investigate the processing mechanisms involved.

It is difficult to make generalisations from these case descriptions. However, it is clear that both semantic and phonological processing must be considered in a child who is presenting with lexical difficulties.

Chapter 2.3
A treatment for anomia combining semantics, phonology and orthography

WENDY BEST, DAVID HOWARD, CAROLYN BRUCE AND CLAIRE GATEHOUSE

Almost everyone with acquired aphasia has difficulties in word retrieval. Over recent years a variety of studies of both individual subjects and groups of patients have investigated the effectiveness of a variety of approaches to treatment (see Nickels and Best 1996a for a review). Howard *et al.* (1985b) drew a distinction between treatment using semantic tasks (e.g. word-to-picture matching) and those that provided information about the phonological form of the word, and demonstrated that both approaches could result in improvements in word retrieval.

These results have since been replicated and extended in a number of ways. Treatment approaches can be broadly categorised into those emphasising access to or use of meaning representations, and those that give information about the spoken or written form of the words. In this introduction, we give examples of these approaches, and discuss briefly how the improvements they cause may be understood in terms of an information processing model of the lexicon.

Semantic treatments

Marshall *et al.* (1990) used an approach where one of four written words had to be matched to a picture, with a group of patients whose reading was better than their naming. This resulted in improvement on the treated items, with more limited improvement on semantically related foils. There was a long-lasting effect from small amounts of treatment (see Pring *et al.* 1990). The finding that improvement generalised to semantically-related items indicates that meaning was important in the treatment. A number of single case studies in which treatment emphasises the meaning of words have also shown improvement in word retrieval (Scott 1987, Jones 1989, Nickels and Best 1996b), and generalisation to related words has frequently been found (Howard *et al.* 1985b, Hillis 1989, Nickels and Best 1996b).

A single case study by LeDorze *et al.* (1994) indicates that semantic treatments may only be effective if the target word is used in therapy. She found that word-to-picture matching improved naming when the subject was asked to find the *octopus* from a choice of semantically-related pictures, but not when asked to find the *mollusc with long arms*. The effect here was, however, not long-lasting.

Lexical treatments

Semantic treatments can be contrasted with those that focus on lexical form. Miceli *et al.* (1994), for example, used three different treatment approaches with a single subject. One involved naming pictures with progressive phonemic cues; the other two required reading the target word aloud with or without the target picture present. All three treatments resulted in item-specific improvement which was maintained. Other single case studies have shown improvement from similar lexical treatments (see Nettleton and Lesser 1991, DF; Hillis and Caramazza 1994, study 2; Nickels and Best 1996b, PA).

Thus, the current information suggests that whereas semantic treatments result in a limited extent of generalisation to related untreated items, the improvements found in lexical therapies are more likely to be limited to the items targeted in treatment. It is also possible, as Hillis and Caramazza (1994) argue, that whether generalisation occurs is related to the nature of the patient's deficit in word retrieval.

Orthographic treatments

A number of researchers have used techniques which mobilise information about the written form of the word in the treatment of difficulties in spoken word retrieval. Berman and Peelle (1967) taught a patient to convert letters into sounds to use knowledge of a word's initial letter to generate a phonemic cue to aid spoken word finding.

Nickels (1992) used a similar technique with a subject, TRC, whose written naming was better than his spoken naming, and who benefited from phonemic cues given by the examiner. She taught him to convert written letters into sounds. He was then able to generate his own phonemic cues. This resulted in his spoken naming improving to the same level as his written naming; the improvement was apparent both with untreated items and in his spontaneous speech.

Bruce and Howard (1987) followed a similar approach using a computerised aid to cue spoken word finding. They worked with five subjects who were able to indicate at greater than chance levels the initial letter of words they could not find in spoken form, and who benefited from phonemic cues given by the examiner. Over five sessions the patients were taught to use a computer-based aid which gave the sounds of letters when their keys were pressed, providing the missing link for self-cueing. After this treatment the patients were better at naming when they could use the aid than where they could not, and the improvement generalised to untreated items. In addition there was a practice effect: pictures involved in treatment were named better than untreated items, even when the cue was not available.

Models of single word processing

The theoretical framework used in considering the assessment and treatment results in this paper is based on the model of Patterson and Shewell (1987) which shows lexical and sub-lexical links between semantic, phonological and orthographic representations (see Figure 2.3.1). The model is elaborated in one respect: Butterworth (1989) and

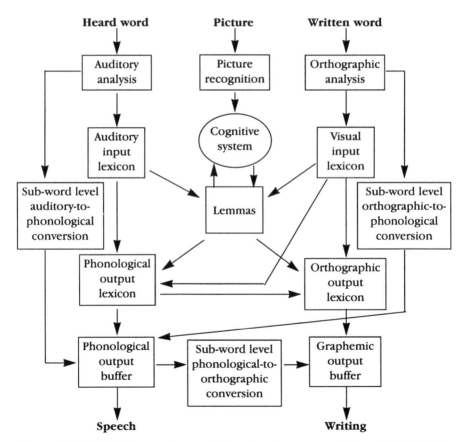

Figure 2.3.1 A lexical processing model based on Patterson and Shewell (1987). This is modified by the addition of a lemma level which intervenes between the input and output lexicons and conceptual semantic information within the cognitive system.

Levelt (1989) among others, have argued that there are two stages in word retrieval. The first stage involves access to an abstract lexical level, which we shall call the **lemma** (using Levelt's term; called a **semantic lexicon** by Butterworth). The second stage involves retrieval of the spoken form of the word within the **phonological output lexicon** (Butterworth's term; the **lexeme** in Levelt). We follow Butterworth *et al.* (1984) and Howard *et al.* (1995) in suggesting that the lemma level is involved in both word production and comprehension. Detailed argument about the form of this model is not appropriate here, but may be found in the cited sources.

This paper describes the outcome of a series of treatments used with a patient with word finding difficulties as result of acquired aphasia. First we describe some pilot studies, and then an experiment contrasting the effects of lexical and semantic treatments. The second treatment study investigates the use of a cueing aid used by Bruce and Howard (1987). In the final section of the paper we briefly sketch the outcome of treatment with the aid with a wider variety of patients.

Subject information

Background

When this study started JOW was 62 years old. He had suffered a left hemisphere CVA 3 years previously in September 1990. There is no scanning information available to localise his lesion.

Previous therapy and presentation at the start of the study

When first seen by a speech and language therapist shortly after his stroke, JOW showed 'high level' comprehension difficulties, and had considerable problems in expressing himself. Over the next year, he had both individual and group speech and language therapy, and in September 1991 he started to attend a general stroke support group for people with dysphasia. JOW's individual treatment in the first year concentrated on helping him to develop and use strategies to overcome his problems with word retrieval, and helping him to communicate more effectively.

When this study began, JOW could understand most everyday conversation, although faster conversation on more abstract topics was problematic. His fluent production was marred by frequent and profound difficulties in word retrieval; when this happened he seemed unable to follow what was said to him. Once blocked on word retrieval he was generally unable to use other strategies, including even responding to forced choice questions, to get his message across. Word finding was hampered by perseveration, often on a specific word which would recur repeatedly within a session, resulting in frustrated rejection of the interloping perseverate.

Employment history and social situation

Before his stroke, JOW had run his own business. At the time of the study, he was in residential care. He seemed more concerned about his social situation than his language impairments. Nevertheless, as we have noted, he found his word retrieval problems frustrating. JOW is hemiplegic, and uses a wheelchair; he needs glasses for reading.

Formal testing

On the Western Aphasia Battery, JOW achieved an aphasia quotient of 69, and was classified as anomic.

Investigations

Here we provide an overview of the findings from the assessments of JOW's language processing. We shall concentrate on his difficulties in word retrieval, as this was the focus both of his concern and of the treatment studies.

Comprehension

JOW was within normal limits on both auditory same–different discrimination, and auditory lexical decision. This suggests that he has no impairment in auditory analysis or in the phonological input lexicon.

On tasks probing semantic ability with concrete items, JOW also scored well. He was 95% correct on the word-to-picture matching tests from PALPA (Kay *et al*. 1992) with both auditory and visual word presentation, and he was within normal limits on the three picture version of the Pyramids and Palm Trees Test (Howard and Patterson 1992).

On comprehension tasks not involving picture stimuli, JOW scored more poorly. He was 79% correct on auditory and 76% correct on visual synonym judgments (from Coltheart 1980). On the three written word version of Pyramids and Palm Trees he was 75% correct. On all these tasks, although JOW scores at a level significantly better than chance, he is substantially below the range of normal control subjects.

To summarise: JOW performed well in more peripheral input tasks, and tasks involving word/picture combinations, but more poorly on semantic tasks involving only words.

Spoken output

Naming

JOW's speech was hampered by word-finding difficulties (see Figure 2.3.2). This difficulty was also evident in picture naming. On a sample of 194 pictures, on which elderly normal controls average 96% correct, JOW named only 28% correctly.

> A tree, a /plæg/, a/mʌ/ er kite theres /bun/ and a girl and a boy and what do you call it? a bicycle, no sorry whats it called? [dog]. A garage and um a /baɪs/ oh [radio] no not a bicycle. [What are they doing?]. They're sat on a bike and pouring out something. He's reading a book. Is that enough?

(a)

> A car in a garage and a bungalow and two fellows, no sorry a boy and a girl sat down eating ... you know ... they eat anything and by the side there's a man flying a kite and a girl, sorry, and a dog and two fellows waving to him and /faɪn/ the yacht. A chap waiting up there, a lake of course. [What else?] A tree over the woods around. I think that's about else.

(b)

Figure 2.3.2 Western Aphasia Battery: picture description (a) pre-treatment, (b) post-treatment. The square brackets contain the therapist's prompt questions and the intended target (*radio*) in (a) determined on the basis of pointing while saying /baɪs/.

Variables affecting picture naming

The effects of a number of variables on picture naming were investigated by generating sub-sets matched on other variables (see Best 1996 for details). He was significantly better at naming items rated high in operativity (i.e. those that are manipulable, firm to the touch, separate from the context and available to several sensory modalities) than those low in operativity (see Howard *et al.* 1995, for further details). He was also better at naming items with higher imageability ratings. Accuracy was not significantly affected by any of the following: word frequency, familiarity, animacy, age of acquisition, or length.

Errors

When JOW was unable to name a target correctly he was rarely able to provide any item-specific information. On 34% of trials he produced no information, 11% of responses included semantic information (e.g. *coffee* → 'Gold cap and here an – um, you know – the brown stuff'), and on a further 8% of trials he rejected his responses. These rejected responses were usually either semantically related or perseverations (e.g. *beard* → 'a man and a bell bicycle [perseveration] Um sorry. He's a ... oh, I lost it'; *daffodil* → '/tu/ no not a tulip, oh um I can't say it'). His remaining responses were classified as visually related (e.g. naming a part of the picture) 5%, phonologically related 2%, and other, including unrelated words and non-words 11%. As well as these spoken responses, JOW sometimes gave rather non-specific gestures to the pictures, few of which would have served to identify the target.

Perseveration

Perseverations were frequent in JOW's naming, and annoying to him. The same word would appear for a number of different pictures, which could be consecutive items or might have intervening correct responses or errors of other kinds. JOW rejected most of these responses at the time, and further perseverations may have been edited out before they actually appeared, where he started his response with '*No!*'.

More detailed analysis of JOW's perseverations showed that 30% were semantically related to the target, which was a level greater than chance. In contrast they showed no reliable tendency to share the same initial phoneme. It seemed that at least some of his perseverations were semantically mediated.

Response to cues

JOW's spoken naming showed a small but significant improvement when given the initial phoneme of the target by the examiner. Further phonological information, in the form of either CV cues or rime cues, resulted in more substantial improvements. He was also helped, significantly, when given the spoken name of the initial letter, but the most substantial improvement was found when he selected the initial letter from one of three written choices.

A miscue – the initial phoneme of a semantically related item -- had no effect on JOW's naming (cf. Howard and Orchard-Lisle 1984).

Serial position effects in naming

JOW was reliably better at naming the first few items in a set than those that occurred later on. This applied both to items occurring at the beginning of a session, or when testing was started after a pause or after a different task. At the start of a block with a 'blank slate' in his production system, his naming was relatively accurate. Then his naming faltered, and no responses, perseverations and semantic errors predominated. This finding was also reflected in JOW's spontaneous speech. He was often able to initiate conversation on a topic but then would get bogged down in unsuccessful word retrieval, and perseverations.

Other output tasks

A subset of 48 items used in the naming test were presented for reading and repetition. There were only two repetition errors, both closely phonologically related to the target. This suggests that his naming problem is unlikely to involve the later stages of speech production which are also necessarily involved in repetition.

His reading accuracy (67%) was significantly better than naming of the same items (38%), but still substantially poorer than repetition. His errors were visual/phonological or perseverations. Whereas in naming he rejected almost all of his perseverations, JOW appeared not to notice them in reading.

A different subset of the 194 items was used for written naming, where JOW was encouraged to write without verbalising his response. His written naming was poor (10% correct) but not significantly worse than spoken naming of the same items. The majority of his errors were no responses. When an attempt was made errors typically contained at least some of the letters in the target (e.g. *piano* → *pancio*). However, errors were never phonologically accurate, suggesting that writing was not phonologically mediated.

Summary and discussion of JOW's naming deficit

JOW's good performance on word-to-picture semantic tasks suggests that he is able to retrieve accurate semantic information from pictures.

A number of lines of evidence suggest that his difficulty is at the lemma level in production. First, both imageability and operativity – variables which are likely to reflect the strength of semantic representations (cf. Plaut and Shallice 1993) – affect JOW's naming accuracy. His principal error types are 'no responses' and semantic errors which probably reflect failures to activate the lemma representations, and activation of semantically related lemmas respectively. The occurrence of perseverations may be related to residual activation at the lemma level, with relatively weak activation of the lemmas by semantics. Where weak semantic activation combines with residual lemma activation, semantically related perseverations result.

Several lines of evidence suggest that more peripheral stages in word retrieval – such as access to phonological forms or phonological assembly – are unlikely to be the source of JOW's naming difficulty. First, his performance is unaffected by frequency or age-of-acquisition, variables associated with the process of access to phonological word forms (e.g. Barry *et al.* in press). Secondly, performance is unaffected by word length, and word production in repetition is excellent. Thirdly, the effect of phonemic cues on word retrieval suggests that he has intact phonological word forms that he fails to activate.

Taken together, this evidence points towards a deficit at the lemma level. Can the problem be more precisely specified? The strong tendency towards perseveration and the serial position effect on naming accuracy suggest that residual activation within the lemma level may overpower the activation of lemmas from semantics. His better naming of high imageability or high operativity targets suggests that these items, which may have richer semantic representations, activate their target lemmas more strongly. As a naming block progresses, residual activation within the lemma level builds up. If there is mutual inhibition within this level, new items will be increasingly inhibited by activation of previous items, with a resulting decline in naming accuracy.

Therapy

Because the major impediment to JOW's conversation and his major concern was the difficulty in word retrieval, this was the focus of our treatment. First we briefly outline the effects of a set of pilot studies. This is followed by more detailed description of two therapy studies. The first contrasts lexical and semantic treatments, and the second describes the results of treatment using the cueing aid.

Pre-therapy assessments and control tasks

The primary way in which we measured the effects of treatment was in spoken picture naming, used because targets can be clearly specified. However, because we were interested in improving his connected spontaneous speech we also assessed his description of a composite picture (from the Western Aphasia Battery) and his description of the room in which treatment took place.

To ensure that any improvement we found was a result of our word finding treatment, we also tested JOW on a number of control tasks. These were neither at ceiling nor at floor levels of performance. We used auditory synonym judgments; although this partly involves concrete word semantics, none of the items involved were targeted in treatment. The second control task was oral reading of single syllable non-words.

Pilot study

Tasks and rationale

We used a variety of different tasks including lexical and semantic treatments which had the potential to influence lemma level processing. The aim was to try out a variety of tasks with the minimum of formal therapy, intending that any that proved effective would be examined in greater depth. As will be seen experimental rigour was neither aimed at nor achieved in these pilot experiments.

The treatments used and the mechanisms which may underlie their effects have been discussed in detail elsewhere (see pp. 102–4). The tasks used in the pilot study are briefly described here.

The semantic task was word-to-picture matching. This was done with a single picture, and a choice of four semantically-related words. JOW had to underline the correct name. This task was done in two ways: in the first no output was required and in the second JOW had to write the picture name after making his selection.

The lexical tasks were similarly ...ied. We describe them as lexical because information was provided about the phonological or ortho-graphic form of the target, and they do not necessarily require semantic processing. JOW was given a set of pictures and asked to try to name each one. If he could not do so, he turned over the card; the target name was written on the back. On different occasions he was asked either to read this name aloud (recall that his oral reading was substan-tially better than his naming), or to write it down.

Finally, a number of other therapy tasks were included. These were:

- reading the name aloud (with no picture present)
- copying of the name on to the back of a card (again with no picture present)
- written naming of the pictures (with the target on the back of the card for checking).

The aim of the pilot study was to compare the effectiveness of these therapy approaches to provide preliminary answers to questions such as:

- Does JOW's naming improve with tasks that require semantic processing?
- Is output of the spoken or written form of the target word helpful in improving his naming?

Method

The set of 194 pictures used for assessment was divided into four subsets, with equal pre-therapy naming accuracy over two sessions. Eight different treatment tasks were used, so each subset was treated twice with different methods. Reassessment on the full set of 194 items followed each of the treatments.

Each task was explained to JOW and a member of the care staff who could practise the task with him. Several practice items were completed during the explanation session. Detailed descriptions of each treatment are given in Best *et al.* (in press). Each of the treatment tasks was prac-tised for one week, except where this proved impossible. Each task was performed between one and three times.

Outcome

Given that the number of times each task was performed varied, we can only consider the results of these pilot studies as indicative.

To summarise, only the written lexical treatment resulted in a signif-icant improvement (from 14 to 27 items correct). Gains were confined to the treated items and were not maintained at the follow-up assessment. There was no significant improvement with any of the other tasks.

A second period of treatment using the written lexical technique again resulted in item-specific improvement (11 to 23 items correct), which this time was sustained for at least two weeks, perhaps because on the second occasion JOW practised each item twice.

This technique, where JOW attempted written naming, and, if unable, copied the name on to the back of a card, helped subsequent spoken naming of the target items. It appears from this that JOW needs both to see the picture (delayed copying alone was ineffective), and to have the target word present (written naming alone did not help).

Discussion

In this pilot study the written lexical treatment improved JOW's spoken naming on two separate occasions even though the practice involved was minimal.

There are two puzzles about the pilot results. First, why should written lexical treatment be effective, but spoken lexical treatment not? It may be that with the spoken version, JOW made errors in reading the words for many items he could not name. Although he made several self-corrections, his writing in the written version was generally accurate. The written task may be more beneficial for another reason: writing takes much longer than speaking and this may result in more sustained activation at the lemma level. It appears that JOW was not slavishly copying the target word because his responses were often in upper case to a lower case model. We will return to this issue later.

The second puzzle is why the semantic treatments were ineffective, including the one involving written output. This treatment had all the elements of written lexical treatment except for the stage of 'trying to name the picture'. It is possible that this is because of the timing of the study. After this semantic treatment, JOW had a severe cold, which delayed reassessment by 9 days. It is possible that there was an effect of this treatment, which was not sustained at the delayed follow-up.

In the first therapy study we therefore decided to re-investigate more formally the effects of a semantic treatment and compare them with written lexical therapy.

Study 1: semantic and lexical therapy

Tasks and rationale

In this experiment we directly compare the effects of written lexical therapy and semantic therapy with written production of the target. The results of the pilot study predicted that written lexical therapy would improve spoken naming, and with a more prolonged period of practice the effects might be longer-lasting. The semantic therapy might prove ineffective, as in the pilot study, or we might find effects when reassessment immediately follows the end of a period of treatment. In addition, we anticipated the possibility of generalised effects from the semantic treatment.

Method

A different set of 72 pictures was used in this experiment. Two baseline assessments were done four weeks apart. The items were randomly divided into two sets with the constraint that baseline accuracy of naming was equal for the two sets. In the written lexical therapy, JOW was presented with pictures from the target set, and asked to write the name of each. When he could not do this, he could use the target name written on the back to help. In the semantic therapy with written output, each target picture was presented with four semantically-related written words which included the target name written on the back of the card in lower case (e.g. apple (target), banana, orange, pear). His task was to underline the target, and then write the name beneath the picture. Each task was attempted six times for each target in separate sessions spread over three weeks.

JOW's spoken naming was assessed on the whole set immediately after each block of treatment, and then 1 month after the second treatment block.

Results

The results are shown in table 2.3.1, and are in marked contrast to the findings of the pilot study. There was no effect of the written lexical treatment. There was an effect of the semantic treatment which generalised to untreated items, but which was not sustained at follow-up. As we pointed out in the introduction, generalisation has been found in a number of previous studies of semantic therapy.

Discussion

With the mismatch between the outcome of this study and the pilot experiments, we might conclude that what is critical in the outcome is not the nature of the tasks involved, but other aspects of the interactions in treatment. From this perspective, without a better theory of therapy (cf. Behrmann and Byng 1993, Caramazza and Hillis 1993, Coltheart *et al.* 1994, Howard and Hatfield 1987) it is unproductive to look in detail at the effects of specific treatments. However, we believe that we can make some progress in understanding this result.

Table 2.3.1 Results of semantic and lexical therapy, number of items correct in each set before and after treatment (*n* = 36 in each set). An asterisk signifies that this set was treated at this point

| | Baselines | | | Post treatment | |
Set	1	2	Lexical	Semantic	Follow-up
1	12	11	9*	22	15
2	13	10	10	23*	13
Total	25	21	19	45	28

Dealing with the effectiveness of the semantic treatment is easier. First, there are indications that multiple repetitions of such treatments are needed for effects lasting long enough to be measurable at the reassessment (Howard *et al.* 1985a, b). Secondly, given that the effects of treatment were no longer apparent at the 1 month follow-up, it is likely that we failed to detect effects in the pilot study because our reassessment was delayed until after JOW had recovered from his cold.

The ineffectiveness of the written lexical treatment in this study may be related to how JOW approached the task. In the pilot study, where the task was novel, he may have carried it out as we planned. In the therapy study where exactly the same procedure was carried out six times, he would have rapidly become aware that the target item was written on the back of the card, and simply and slavishly copied the item. We have some evidence in support of this conjecture which comes from the case of his written responses in this task.

Almost all of JOW's spontaneous writing was in upper case, while the written words offered for copying were in lower case. We would, therefore, anticipate that lower case copies are more likely to involve slavish reproduction, while upper case responses are more likely to stem from involvement of lexical processes. We therefore compared the case of his written responses in the pilot study and in this experiment. In the pilot study 40% of his responses were wholly in upper case. In this experiment the proportion fell to 18% – a highly significant difference (χ^2 (1)=20.53, p < 0.001). This evidence suggests that in the pilot study JOW was performing the task differently with more lexical involvement.

In summary, this experiment showed that a therapy task which involved semantic processing resulted in generalised improvement in naming which lasted for less than four weeks. The written lexical therapy, in contrast to the pilot study, resulted in no improvement, probably because JOW slavishly copied the target words.

Study 2: cueing aid therapy

Rationale

Bruce and Howard (1987) showed that treatment with a cueing aid was effective for subjects who both knew about the initial letters of words they could not produce and benefited from initial phoneme cues in spoken naming. The aid then provides the missing link in allowing patients to turn their initial letter knowledge into a phonemic cue. JOW was a potential candidate for this approach to treatment. He showed a small, but significant, degree of benefit from phonemic cues, and when given a choice of 3 possible initial letters his spoken naming improved. However, when given a choice of 10 possible initial letters, he was no better than chance in choosing the right one.

The cueing aid consisted of a A5 sized box. There was a keyboard restricted to nine possible letters; when a key was pressed the corresponding phoneme, followed by schwa, was produced.

Method

As a baseline JOW named the set of 194 items on three occasions. The set of 190 items beginning with nine different initial letters was the focus of therapy. First we selected the 100 items with least successful naming over the baseline tests and randomly assigned these to the treatment and control sets, with the constraint of equal baseline performance on the two sets. A further set of the 50 most successful items in the baseline ('fillers'), were also used in treatment.

The control items were to see whether improvement with the aid would generalise to a set of items with the same initial letters. We also tested JOW pre-treatment on a set of 32 items with different initial letters so that we could examine whether improvements generalised to pictures with other initial letters.

Treatment took place in five weekly sessions. In the first three sessions, JOW was required to use the aid before attempting to name the pictures; in the last two sessions he could choose to use the aid when he wished. In each session all the treatment items and fillers were presented once in random order.

The treatment followed the same sequence when each picture was presented:

1. Press the initial letter (if failed/incorrect go to step 4).
2. Repeat the cue given by the aid
3. Name the picture (if incorrect go to step 5; otherwise stop).
4. Therapist restricts the choice to three letters; go to step 1.
5. Therapist says the name; patient repeats it. Stop.

After treatment, JOW's naming of the complete set was reassessed with and without the cueing aid available, over two sessions a week apart, with half the items in each session tested with the aid and half without. Reassessment of naming without the aid available followed 5 weeks and 15 months later.

Response during treatment

JOW participated willingly in the treatment sessions, and the incidence of perseveration in his naming was much reduced. However, he expressed no more enthusiasm for this treatment than the others which had preceded it. His naming accuracy during the treatment sessions is shown in table 2.3.2. The number of items JOW named without the therapist's intervention increased substantially after the first session (from 23 to 48%); after that there was little change.

Table 2.3.2 Naming during treatment sessions, in relation to the step in the treatment schedule given in the text ($n = 100$)

Session	Named alone	Named with help (step 4)	Total
1	23	17	40
2	48	13	61
3	47	12	59
4	54	17	71
5	51	14	65

Results: post-therapy assessments

The baseline naming and the results of assessment at the end of treatment are shown in table 2.3.3. On the whole set, JOW improves from a baseline mean of 34% to 48% correct naming without a cue. Improvement is significant on the set of items taken as a whole (Wilcoxon, $z = 3.90$, $p < 0.001$), and significant for the treated items (Wilcoxon, $z = 3.92$, $p < 0.001$), the controls ($z = 3.23$, $p < 0.001$) and the others ($z = 2.11$, $p < 0.02$). The degree of improvement on the treated items and the controls is equal indicating that there has been complete generalisation of improvement to untreated control items.

However, JOW was not helped by using the aid; naming with the aid after treatment (55%) was marginally, but not significantly, better than naming unaided (48%; McNemar's test, $p < 0.09$). Thus training in using the aid improved JOW's word retrieval, although he did not benefit from using the aid as a prosthesis.

The set of pictures with names with different initial letters was used to investigate whether improvement generalised to all initial letters.

Table 2.3.3 Naming before and after treatment with the cueing aid (proportion correct)

| | Baseline | | | | Post-treatment | |
	1	2	3	Mean	With aid	No aid
Treated	0.08	0.10	0.06	0.08	0.40	0.38
Controls	0.08	0.10	0.06	0.08	0.40	0.30
Fillers	0.76	0.74	0.84	0.78	0.84	0.68
Others	0.33	0.53	0.48	0.44	0.55	0.60
Total	0.31	0.36	0.35	0.34	0.55	0.48

With this set, JOW named 25% correctly pre-therapy and 50% post-therapy, a significant difference (McNemar's test, $p < 0.04$). Improvement with this set is equivalent to that in the main assessment set.

Follow-up

Semantic therapy in our first experiment resulted in substantial and generalised improvement, which had disappeared at follow-up 4 weeks later. Are the improvements from aid therapy sustained? At immediate reassessment JOW named 48% of the items unaided. On presentation of the complete set 5 weeks later he named 53%, and 15 months later he named 55%. The effects of this treatment were sustained for over a year.

Figure 2.3.3 shows JOW's naming accuracy with the complete set of 194 items on a series of occasions spanning from the beginning of the pilot study to the final follow-up 15 months after the end of the cueing therapy. This shows that the effect of this treatment was both decisive and long-lasting.

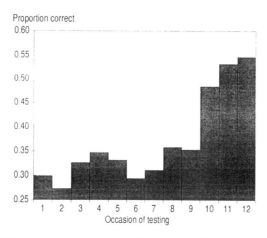

Figure 2.3.3 JOW's naming accuracy on the set of 194 items from the beginning of the pilot studies (testing session 1), to the pre-aid therapy baselines (sessions 7, 8 and 9), with immediate reassessment (session 10), 5 week follow-up (session 11) and 15 month follow-up (session 12).

Connected speech

We wished to establish whether the improvement evident in picture naming could also be found in his spontaneous speech. JOW said that he had benefited from the aid therapy, but he had shown similar degrees of enthusiasm about the other treatments that had had no long-lasting effects

Assessment of improvement in spontaneous speech can be problematic (Lesser and Milroy 1993). After treatment there was an increase in the number of content words used in picture description (from 13/52 to 22/73; see Figure 2.3.2). To analyse the change in spontaneous speech quality in JOW's description of the room in which he was seen, we used a rating procedure based on LeDorze *et al.* (1994). Audio recordings of both samples were rated by eight experienced speech and language therapists, on:

• the patient's ability to transmit the message
• his ability to find adequate words.

(LeDorze *et al.* (1994) also gathered ratings of the quantity of information contained in the sample. This was not possible for JOW as the room he was describing had changed. Before treatment the room contained a large cabinet with a variety of ornaments on the shelves. But, before the reassessment after treatment, a royal visit left the room redecorated but bare of the cabinet and ornaments so usefully present beforehand. A lack of change in the quantity of information from pre- to post- therapy could simply reflect the lack of items on which to comment.)

The raters were blind to whether samples were from before or after treatment, and the order of the samples was counterbalanced across raters; both aspects were rated on a 0–5 scale. The mean rating for ability to transfer the message improved from 0.47 (sd 0.31) to 2.21 (sd 0.85) – a highly significant improvement ($t(7)=9.11$, $p < 0.001$). Similar improvement was found in ratings of word finding from 0.72 (sd 0.29) pre-treatment to 2.66 (sd 0.77) post-treatment – again the improvement was highly significant ($t(7)= 11.43, p < 0.001$).

Control tasks

The improvement found with the aid therapy showed complete generalisation to untreated items. This result is compatible with a generalised effect of treatment, but it is also compatible with a quite general improvement in language function which occurred coincidentally with this therapy. To evaluate this we reassessed JOW on the control tasks. If the improvement is a specific result of the treatment used aimed at word retrieval, there should be no change in the control tasks. A general improvement in language function unrelated to the treatment should result in improvement in the control tasks as well.

The results are shown in table 2.3.4. There are no significant changes in synonym judgement accuracy or in non-word reading over the course of this treatment. This gives us confidence that JOW's improvement was truly a treatment effect.

Table 2.3.4 Control task performance, before treatment, after lexical and semantic treatments and after treatment with the aid

Task	Pre-treatment 1	Pre-treatment 2	Post lexical and semantic treatments	Post-treatment with cueing aid
Synonym judgements ($n = 76$)				
High imageability	31	31	34	36
Low imageability	29	27	30	26
Overall proportion correct	0.77	0.76	0.82	0.79
Non-word reading ($n = 25$)	8	not tested	10	8

Related tasks

Two further tasks were tested before any treatment and again after the conclusion of the aid therapy. These are both functions related to the aid treatment, and the results are presented here for the light they may cast on how and why JOW improved.

On the first task, letter-to-sound conversion, JOW improved substantially. Before treatment he could give a correct sound to 2/20 written letters; after the aid therapy he could do so for 13/20 – a highly significant difference (McNemar, $p < 0.001$). The change applied both to items involved in treatment and those that were not. He tended to do this task using an overt lexical relay strategy (cf. de Partz 1986); his improvement in this task may reflect improvements in initial sound segmentation. Before treatment, given the letter R, he said 'ram, ram, no is it?' After aid therapy he said 'rabbit, um /rə/'. Although the therapy never explicitly targeted segmentation skills, it did involve repeated identification of initial letters and repetition of their sounds given by the aid, emphasising the letter–sound relationship.

The second related task was written naming. When testing this we encouraged JOW to write without saying the word first. Before therapy he wrote 5/48 names correctly, and after treatment 4/48. As the therapy emphasised knowledge of initial letters we examined whether his accuracy in writing initial letters had improved. Pre-therapy 13 of his errors had the correct initial letter; post-treatment 17 did. It is clear from this that there was no significant improvement in JOW's written naming or in his knowledge of initial letters in the course of treatment.

Discussion

As figure 2.3.3 illustrates, while the previous therapies had had little impact on JOW's word-finding difficulties, the treatment with the aid resulted in substantial and long-lasting improvement. The improvement was equal for items involved in treatment and those that were not; that is, there was perfect generalisation of the treatment effects. There was no change in performance in the control tasks. Therefore the effects cannot be attributed to spontaneous recovery. Moreover, given that JOW had been seen for extended periods and treated with a variety of methods, the improvement with aid therapy cannot be attributed to practice effects or any other kinds of non-specific effects of treatment.

Here we discuss how the aid therapy might have improved JOW's word retrieval. We will consider three possible accounts: lexical priming, sub-lexical cueing and lexical cueing.

Lexical priming
The effects of treatment may be due to priming at the level of the lemmas (cf. Howard *et al.* 1985a). If, as we have argued, JOW has a deficit in access to the lemma representations, repeated presentation of the items during treatment might result in increased ease of access to the lemmas of treated words, resulting in improved naming post-therapy. On this account the treatment may have been working in the same way as the lexical treatment in the pilot study. This account can, however, be immediately rejected as it should predict item-specific improvement, and cannot explain the generalisation to items not involved in treatment.

Sub-lexical cueing
Nickels (1992) treated her patient TRC by enabling him to use his knowledge of initial letters to internally (or in some cases overtly) generate his own phonemic cues. Could JOW have acquired this mechanism?

There is some attractiveness in this proposal. Before treatment JOW benefited from phonemic cues, and may have had some knowledge of words' initial letters. Also, after treatment his knowledge of letter–sound relationships was much improved.

There are, however, two reasons why we think this account is unlikely to be correct. First, JOW's letter-to-sound conversion, while significantly improved in accuracy, remained slow and dependent on lexical processing (thinking of a word with that initial letter and then segmenting off the first sound). Second, at no point were there any overt signs of JOW using this strategy, although he explicitly used it in letter–sound conversion. He never said letter names; he never said initial phonemes; he never finger-wrote initial letters in the air or on a table. Furthermore his written naming, and his ability to write the first letter of a target word did not change during treatment. If he were using this method of self-cueing one would have to conclude that it was completely internalised and implicit. Given that previous accounts of patients using this kind of strategy have shown that developing any kind of automaticity in the process takes a great deal of therapy (cf. Berman and Peelle 1967, de Partz 1986, Nickels 1992) it seems implausible that five sessions at weekly intervals were sufficient to establish such a procedure.

The other question this account raises is at a theoretical level. It is generally agreed that phonemic cues operate by combined information from the cue and from semantics summating to make a word available for output (see Howard and Orchard-Lisle 1984, Ellis 1985, Monsell 1987). What is less clear is where this summation might occur. The lexical model in figure 2.3.1 supposes that sub-lexical grapheme to phoneme conversion yields a phoneme held in the phonological output buffer. A variety of sources of evidence suggest that there is feedback from this level to the phonological output lexicon (e.g. Howard and Franklin 1990, Martin *et al.* 1994, Hillis and Caramazza 1995, Best 1996). Sub-threshold activation from semantics to the phonological output lexicon combines with the feedback from the output buffer to the lexicon, to elicit the appropriate item for output. This mechanism would work for a model with a single stage of phonological output. We argued, however, that JOW's impairment could be most satisfactorily explained by a deficit at the level of the lemma. To sustain an account of this kind we would need either to suppose a cascade of partial information through the lemma level to the phonological output lexicon, or feedback from the lexical level to the lemma.

Lexical cueing
The final possibility that we want to consider is that the treatment has enabled JOW to use orthographic knowledge directly to aid his spoken word retrieval, by a routine that does not involve implicit or explicit grapheme-to-phoneme conversion.

A patient described by Harding (1993) illustrates how this might work. This subject, SD, improved dramatically in naming when she could use a letter board to identify the initial letter of a word. Although SD benefitted from phonemic cues given by the experimenter, Harding argues that this cannot account for the letter board cueing effect. This is because SD was completely unable to convert letters into sounds – she was, in fact, deep dyslexic in reading. Harding argues that the initial letter activates a cohort of items in a visual input lexicon. Activation from these lexical entries cascades to the phonological output lexicon via the direct, non-semantic route shown in Figure 2.3.1. Activation of the correct phonological item from the semantics of the picture is insufficient to activate the appropriate output lexicon entry to threshold. When it is combined with the partial activation from the visual input lexicon, this is sufficient to allow production of the correct word.

During the aid therapy, JOW was required to identify the initial letter of the words and to try to use this information to aid word retrieval. His responses in letter-to-sound conversion before treatment suggest that he could use a single letter to activate words' representations for phonological output. Moreover, his naming pre-therapy improved when given a choice of three possible initial letters of the name. In written naming he could write at least the initial letter of a target on 31% of occasions. Pre-treatment he was correct in naming 34% of items. If, after therapy he has become able to use his initial letter knowledge (available for 31% of items) to improve his naming of the 66% of items he would otherwise be unable to name, we would predict that he would be able to name an additional (31% $\times$ 66%) = 20% of items. This prediction corresponds almost exactly to the 20% improvement in naming he actually made in the course of treatment.

This hypothesis is that the treatment with the aid has allowed JOW to use a set of sources of information which he had available before therapy to orthographically cue his written naming. The question that this raises is why, if the information was available pre-therapy, was the treatment necessary? We suggest that the reason is that the aid explicitly required JOW to use partial orthographic knowledge to aid word finding, and the aid itself drew attention to the systematic relationship between a letter and its sound, and the use of that information in word retrieval. The aid, by requiring him to put these separate skills together, enabled him to make the link. This linking, however, is different in kind from the conscious and deliberate ways in which orthography has been used to improve word retrieval by, for instance, de Partz (1986) and Nickels (1992); instead the treatment has effected a fundamental change in the way JOW's word retrieval operates, altering automatic and not strategic processes in his linguistic system.

Note that this account requires summation of partial information about the phonology of the target with sub-threshold activation from semantics. Just as with the account in terms of self-generated cues we need to argue that, if JOW has a lemma level of deficit, there is a locus at which this summation of activation can occur. If summation is at the level of the phonological output lexicon, we have to posit a cascade of partial information from the lemma level to the phonological lexicon. If summation is taking place at the lemma level there must be feedback from the level of the phonological lexicon to the lemmas. Feedback of this kind is suggested by a number of authors to account for some aspects of speech errors in normals (see for example Dell 1986, 1989, Harley and MacAndrew 1992, Levelt 1992). A possible architecture, which is consistent with these interpretations and the other sources of evidence is shown in figure 2.3.4.

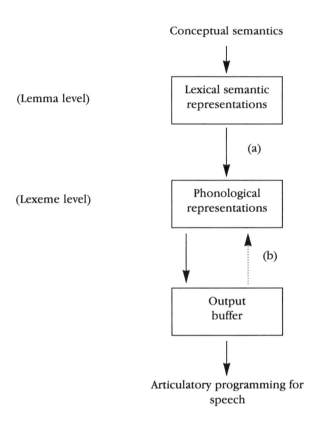

Figure 2.3.4 A two stage model of word retrieval with interaction between the output buffer and the output lexicon (b). To explain JOW's results we must suppose that the connection at (a) either allows a cascade of partial information or that there is feedback from the phonological lexicon to the lemma level.

The effects of cueing aid therapy with other aphasic patients

The results from JOW show that, although he did not benefit directly from the aid, in that his naming performance after treatment was no better when he was able to use it than when he was not, the treatment caused highly significant and long-lasting improvement in word retrieval which generalised from items involved in therapy to control items which were never seen during treatment.

JOW was, in fact, one of 13 aphasic patients who were treated with the cueing aid adopting the same experimental design. In this section of the paper we present the data from all 13 patients to explore the extent to which this pattern of improvement is found with other aphasic patients.

Method

The patients involved had chronic aphasia (all were at least 6 months post-onset) with significant degrees of impairment in word retrieval. These patients varied in their ability to benefit from therapist-given initial phoneme cues, and in their ability to indicate the initial letter of words which they could not produce. In accordance with Bruce and Howard (1987), we predicted that benefits from using the aid should be found only with patients who both benefited from phonemic cues and knew the identity of initial letters of names they could not produce. Only two of the subjects were significantly different from chance in both of these functions. We therefore predicted that, after learning to use the cueing aid, only these two subjects were likely to be better at naming when using the aid than with unaided naming. The other patients were not likely to benefit directly from the cueing aid.

The design of the treatment study was essentially the same for these 12 additional patients as for JOW. Before therapy, patients were assessed in naming the set of 190 items in three sessions. The first two sessions were separated by at least 1 month, and the third pre-therapy session followed immediately before treatment began. The interval between the first two sessions was filled with weekly assessment sessions involving other aspects of their performance, not reported in detail here. This period between the first two sessions, which involved contact with a therapist and attention, thus serves as a control for improvements found over an equivalent period with treatment.

After the third pre-therapy assessment, items were selected for treatment. The 100 items which had the lowest overall accuracy in the three pre-tests were assigned to two equal sets such that the mean correct naming was equal for both sets in the three pre-tests. The two sets were then randomly assigned to treatment and control conditions. The comparison between these two sets in post-therapy naming can be used to assess generalisation; item-specific improvements should result in better naming of treatment items than controls, but if improvement generalises there should be no significant differences between the two sets. The 50 items which were named most accurately over the three pre-tests served as filler items during treatment.

There then followed five weekly treatment sessions involving the 50 treatment items and 50 fillers, in exactly the same format as we used with JOW. One week after the final treatment session the whole set was again presented for naming; in this session half the items were presented with the cueing aid available, and the patients were encouraged to use it whenever they thought it was helpful. The remaining items were presented for unaided naming. A week later the same items were presented, and the availability of the cue reversed (again using an ABAB and BABA design). Thus over these two sessions each item was presented both with and without the aid. Comparison between these conditions allows us to assess the extent to which patients benefit from using the cueing aid. Comparison of unaided naming with performance in the three pre-tests measures the extent to which naming has benefited from the treatment. A final naming session followed 5 weeks later: the whole set were presented for naming without the aid. This gives us a measure of the stability of any improvements in name retrieval.

Results

While acknowledging that the patterns of results show substantial inter-subject variation, in this section we will, for reasons of space, only present the average results across the 13 subjects; this is to indicate the extent to which JOW's pattern of improvement in aid therapy holds for the other subjects.

Usefulness of the cueing aid after treatment

Across all the patients, naming with the aid was marginally less accurate than unaided naming (57% vs 59%). The difference was not significant ($t(12) = 0.72$, ns). In fact only one subject, who was one of the two patients where we anticipated the aid might be helpful, showed any effect of the aid being present after treatment. He was reliably better at naming with the aid than without, but only when given 20 seconds to produce a response, and this effect was confined to the items involved in treatment.

Improvement in treatment

Taking the 13 patients as a group, mean naming accuracy increases from 47% over the three pre-tests to 59% in the unaided post-test, and 56% 5 weeks later (see Figure 2.3.5). An analysis of variance on the scores over the five tests shows significant differences ($F(4,48) = 15.78, p < 0.001$). Conservative posthoc tests using Tukey's honestly significant difference show that both post-tests are reliably better than all three pre-tests and do not differ significantly from each other. The second pre-test (carried out during the baseline testing) is also just significantly better than the first, suggesting that at least some of the patients may have benefited from the assessment and attention that filled the interval between these tests.

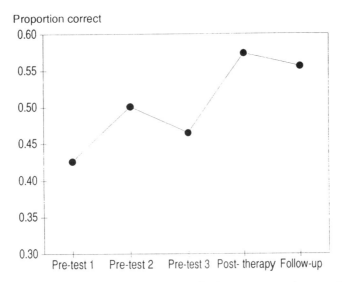

Figure 2.3.5 The mean naming accuracy of 13 patients on the set of 194 items before and after treatment with the cueing aid.

The results from the patients as a group, therefore, mirror those of JOW. There was improvement as a result of learning to use the aid, with improvement sustained to the 5 week follow up.

Generalisation of improvement to untreated items

Overall improvement can only be given an unbiased assessment on the basis of performance on the whole set. Generalisation of improvement, on the other hand, can only be tested by comparing naming of the 50 treated items and the 50 untreated controls at the post-therapy tests.

Figure 2.3.6 shows the mean performance of the 13 patients on the treated and control items. Analysis of variance on the scores of treated and control items post-therapy and at reassessment shows overall better naming of the treated items than controls $(F(1,12)=8.53, p = 0.013)$, but no significant effect of session $(F(1,12)=4.10, p = 0.066)$ and no interaction between item type and test session $(F(1,12)=3.80, p = 0.075)$. This indicates that there was better naming of the treated items than the controls, but this difference was stable over the testing sessions.

Individually, the patients showed varied patterns. Some subjects, like JOW, showed complete generalisation of improvement with no significant difference in naming accuracy with treated items and controls. Some subjects showed item-specific benefits from treatment, and some subjects showed no unequivocal evidence that they benefited from treatment.

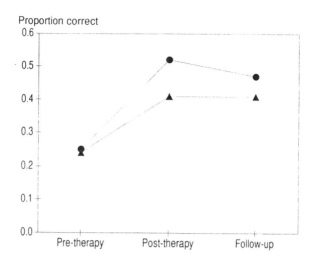

Figure 2.3.6 The mean naming accuracy of 13 patients on the treated items (black circle) and untreated controls (black triangles) before and after treatment with the cueing aid (*n* = 50 of each type).

General discussion

JOW showed substantial and long-lasting effects of learning to use the cueing aid, which generalised to untreated items. The beneficial effect of aid treatment was also found for these patients as a group, and it was sustained to follow-up. The group results, on the other hand, show significantly greater improvement with treated items than control items.

Clearly this treatment, although very small in amount, caused significant changes in ability to name pictures in many of the patients who took part. Only two patients, however, had the abilities which would make us think that they might benefit from learning to use the aid. And, as it turned out, only one subject was better at naming when using the cueing aid. This leaves us with a paradox: most patients did not appear to have the abilities to use the aid, and, even after treatment, were unable to benefit from its presence. Why then did treatment with the aid result in substantial improvements in naming?

Recent connectionist models may provide some help in understanding this result. Allport (1985) and Farah and McClelland (1991) have proposed that lexical representations may consist of distributed patterns of activation across semantic, orthographic and phonological domains. Within these interactive networks, activation of a representation within one domain will tend to evoke the representations within the other. In general, co-activation of parts of representations will tend to strengthen the connections between them. From this perspective, the critical part of our treatment is that it involves simultaneous activation of phonological, semantic and orthographic representations. The more the representations are evoked together the more strongly they will be linked and then this strengthened representation will be more easily evoked. Thus the treatment may result in improved word retrieval for treated items. Plaut's recent simulations suggest that at least within some connectionist models there may be generalisation of treatment effects to other untreated items (Plaut, 1996). The extent to which generalisation will be found across connectionist models of different kinds of architectures remains to be clarified, but it is clear that generalisation of improvement should be found under some circumstances (see Coltheart and Byng 1989).

Although these proposals provide at least a sketch of why the treatment involved in this study may have benefited the patients, there are many important questions which cannot be addressed without much more detailed models. Patients varied in the degree to which they improved; they varied in the extent to which improvement was sustained after therapy was over; and they varied in the extent to which improvement was confined to the treated items or generalised to untreated controls. Understanding the sources of such variation is, of course, critical in deciding whether a particular type of treatment should be given to an individual patient. We should also acknowledge that the different patients in the cueing study may have improved for different reasons. We argued that JOW benefited because he developed a direct orthographic cueing mechanism. Other subjects may have used sub-lexical cueing, and others may have improved because of a general strengthening of connections within distributed networks.

The results of this study are encouraging. The amount of treatment was small; only 50 hard-to-name items were treated (together with 50 easy-to-name fillers). Each of these was named only once in each of five weekly sessions, yet substantial improvements could be detected on the immediate post-therapy assessments (1–2 weeks after the end of treatment) and at the follow-up five weeks later. And, at least in JOW's case, these effects were still apparent 1 year after treatment (the relevant data were not collected for the other subjects).

In devising selection criteria for patients to be given this, or similar treatment, several points come from the investigations with JOW. Patients do not necessarily have to benefit dramatically from phonemic cues. Their written naming does not have to be better than spoken naming; however, some orthographic knowledge may be useful. JOW was sometimes able to find the initial letter when unable to produce the spoken name and his word finding benefited from being provided with a choice of three written letters. Treatment may have allowed JOW to make use of this limited orthographic information in a way that dramatically improved his spoken naming.

Although the different treatments used with JOW were not matched for the amount of direct involvement of the therapist in the treatment (there was more contact time with the cueing aid therapy), even the time spent on the treatment with the aid was relatively small (five sessions of approximately 1 hour) and, in fact, the majority of improvement may have occurred within a single session of treatment (see Table 2.3.2).

The results suggest that even when a patient is a long time post-onset and has received a considerable amount of other treatment it may be worth treating using the cueing aid. As long as the treatment is being evaluated, with the short time taken by the treatment, the potential benefits to untreated and treated items and more importantly potential generalisation to connected speech, there is little to lose. In addition, in relation to financial constraints which might prevent such an aid being available on a long term basis, JOW did not need the aid to be present to find words after treatment.

Acknowledgments

We thank JOW and the other aphasic people for their participation in this research. This work was supported by grants from the Stroke Association and the Medical Research Council.

Chapter 2.4
Afterword

JANE MARSHALL

Drawing comparisons between the cases in this section is difficult. The studies were carried out independently of one another and, as a result, used quite different assessment and therapy techniques. They also varied considerably in their nature and design. We can therefore only draw tentative conclusions.

The first issue to consider is whether the word finding problems experienced by the individuals originated from similar or different processing deficits. Clearly there were similarities. All three showed good peripheral speech skills. For example, they could all repeat well, and much better than they could name (Richard had difficulty repeating non-words, but this is attributed to input problems). We can therefore be fairly confident that their poor word finding had little to do with low level speech production problems.

Another point of comparison was in the subjects' semantic skills, in that all three showed some weakness at this level. Taking JOW first, he could only succeed on semantic tasks if pictures were involved. In purely lexical tasks, such as synonym judgement, errors were made. Furthermore his naming was influenced by semantic variables, such as imageability and operability and he was more likely to perseverate on a word if that word bore some semantic relationship to the target. Best *et al.* conclude that his key deficit lay at the lexical-semantic level. Richard and Rosie also showed semantic problems. They produced semantic errors in their speech and, when asked to judge picture names, accepted semantic correlates as correct. Like children with normally developing language, they could formulate associations between pictures, but, unlike 'normals', found it difficult to explain and elaborate upon those associations.

The fact that all three patients made errors on semantic tests does not, of course, allow us to conclude that they had the same deficit, particularly as the tests in question varied. Best *et al.* argue that JOW's deficit was primarily one of access, rather than a loss of representations.

They cite in evidence his positive response to cues and the variability in his naming, i.e. an item which was not achieved on one occasion might be on the next. They also speculate that the access problem was exacerbated by slow decay rates. The evidence for this was his perseveration. Thus words which he had produced on a previous occasion remained partially activated. These lingering words were likely to intrude as perseverations, particularly if JOW subsequently targeted a related item. Lewis and Speake are less specific about the nature of Richard and Rosie's problems. However, in both cases, they suggest that the deficit was not simply one of access. In addition, the representations themselves were impoverished. This impoverishment may have taken two forms. Firstly, Lewis and Speake argue that known words were not fully specified. As a result, in the semantic links task, both children found it difficult to generate the normal range of associations between the related pictures. Secondly, representations for some items were entirely missing, as was evidenced by their delayed vocabulary acquisition. (In Rosie's case we cannot explain this by appealing to her bilingualism, since her problems in Cantonese were apparently similar.)

These accounts of the patients' deficits remain speculative. However, we might reflect upon the different consequences of an acquired as opposed to a developmental semantic impairment. JOW once had a normal semantic system. It is perfectly feasible that an impairment could block access to that system, without necessarily disrupting the representations within it. In contrast, Richard and Rosie's impairment occurred in the context of language acquisition. It seems almost inevitable that this impairment would disrupt their ability to lay down fully specified semantic representations, as well as impeding access to those representations. Furthermore, we might predict that some aspects of semantics may be more fully developed than others. For example, perceptual semantic features, which are partly derived from sensory motor experiences, may be quite fully developed, whereas more abstract features may not. However, without more in-depth exploration of the semantic processing that each child could achieve, it is difficult to pursue these ideas much further.

Turning to phonology, this aspect of processing clearly varied between the three subjects. JOW showed no input difficulties, i.e. his auditory discrimination, repetition and lexical decision were good. His response to phonological cues also suggested that output phonological representations were retained, although he often failed to access them. Comparisons with Richard and Rosie are problematic, as they were tested on different measures. However, it seems that Rosie shared JOW's input strengths, since she had good discrimination and repetition skills. She was also able to reflect upon her internal phonological representations. For example, she could judge the first sounds of words and decide whether the names of pictures rhymed. Richard's phonological skills were much less intact. He showed input difficulties with novel phonological material and was much poorer than Rosie on first phoneme and rhyme tasks. It is difficult to judge the contribution of Richard's phonological impairment to his naming deficit. Interestingly, he could apparently exploit lexical and semantic knowledge to help him overcome some of these difficulties on input. Thus his discrimination and repetition of words was much better than his discrimination and repetition of non-words. However, this was apparently not possible on output.

We can conclude that, while there were some processing similarities, the lexical problems of these three subjects were clearly quite different. Furthermore, any possible similarities have to be qualified by the insensitivity of our tests and the probably very different functional consequences of acquired as opposed to developmental deficits.

The second issue we would like to consider is how the diagnosed deficits of the three cases related to the content and outcome of their therapies. In all three cases the links are quite obscure. JOW's main deficit was semantic, which suggested that he would require therapy that involved some degree of semantic processing. However, in the pilot study he made most progress with the written lexical treatment, which simply encouraged him to write the name of a picture with a written model on the back. Confusingly, this result was not replicated. Instead, in the subsequent therapy study he gained most from the semantic treatment, although the results were not maintained. Finally the cueing aid was attempted. Arguably, the prognosis for success with the aid was quite poor. Firstly, JOW was unable to chose the first letter of a word from an array of 10, which suggested that he would find it difficult to use the aid. Secondly, the previous therapy study indicated that he was most likely to profit from a treatment which included a semantic element, which was not the case for the cueing aid therapy. Despite this, he made rapid and startling progress. Furthermore the effects of the therapy were still evident 15 months after it had ceased.

Best *et al.* make a valiant attempt to account for these apparently contradictory results. In the case of the pilot and the first therapy study they speculate that JOW's approach to the tasks was crucial. Taking the evidence of the written case used by JOW, they argue that in the pilot programme he made a genuine attempt to name the pictures in the lexical treatment, whereas in the subsequent therapy study he merely copied the provided name. This is an excellent and perceptive point. It reminds us that one of the many imponderables of therapy is how the person uses the task. In some cases, as with JOW, the patient may provide us with some hints about this, while in others we are left guessing.

When trying to explain the effects of the cueing aid, Best *et al.* draw upon a number of related tasks. After therapy, JOW was no better at written naming, even in terms of his ability to access the first letter of a word. This suggested that he did not use the aid to develop a strategy, in which he accessed the first letter of a word and then converted it into a phonological cue. Instead, the authors argue that the aid enabled him to make more effective use of the orthographic skills which were already available to him. This is the story JOW uses his knowledge about the first letter of the word in order partially to activate the input orthographic representations of all words starting with that letter. This activation is relayed to the phonological output lexicon, via direct input to output connections. The output lexicon also receives partial semantic activation from the picture. These two sources of activation, in combination, are enough to access the target.

In discussing the group study, Best *et al.* again argue that the aid has the potential to activate different levels of representation within the lexical system and hence to strengthen access to the target. Taken to its logical conclusion, this argument suggests that virtually any information we give a patient about a blocked word (be it orthographic, semantic or phonological) might help to elicit its production. In other words, it sounds rather like a call for multimodal stimulation. This, in turn, suggests that detailed investigations of the processes which are or are not available to patients might be rather redundant in the context of therapy planning. Providing we give the person enough varied exposure to a word, something will happen. However, whether or not stimulation is effective is, of course, dependent on whether the person can process that stimulation. The cueing aid might have helped JOW because it tapped into his residual orthographic skills. The group subjects may have drawn upon different skills in their system.

Turning to Richard and Rosie, assessment showed that the children had quite different processing skills, particularly in terms of phonology. However, quite similar therapies were attempted. Lewis and Speake argue that, although the tasks were similar, the rationales varied. Thus Richard's therapy, in part, aimed to strengthen phonological representations, while Rosie's aimed to improve semantic access partly by exploiting her already good phonological skills.

In conclusion, we shall suggest some possible new directions for further research.

If we are to conduct future comparative studies between children and adults we clearly need to apply similar methodologies. In terms of assessment, this would require the creation of tasks which can either be administered to both children and adults, or which are at least underpinned by the same theoretical assumptions. This might be accomplished by creating a 'developmental PALPA', with tasks which parallel the current battery, although with age appropriate stimuli and developmental norms. Once parallel assessments are available, we can begin to explore how particular processing deficits manifest in the developmental as opposed to the acquired domain. In particular, we might anticipate that developmental deficits will impede the establishment of lexical representations, as well as access to them. There may also be fewer clear cut dissociations in childhood disorders, since impairments at one level of a developing system may necessarily affect processing at another.

Parallel approaches could also be applied in therapy. In other words, we might aim to administer therapies which tap similar levels of processing, although with age adapted materials and methods. Part of the endeavour here would be to see if roughly the same therapies work for the same types of processing problem, regardless of whether we are treating an adult or child. We might also explore more qualitative aspects of therapy, like how children and adults tackle a therapy task, and whether or not they use it to develop similar strategies.

Finally, we need to apply parallel methods of evaluation. In the acquired domain, the use of experimental methodology to evaluate therapy is now familiar, although it may not be applied routinely in clinic. The approach is perhaps less developed in the paediatric domain. This is possibly because of the particular problems involved in evaluating therapy with children. Unlike people with acquired problems, children are still maturing. Therefore we cannot depend upon a stable baseline. Furthermore, their speech and language therapy occurs alongside the full educational curriculum, which, hopefully, also brings about changes. Therefore, selecting control tasks which will remain unchanged during the therapy period is likely to be problematic. Despite these challenges, it seems essential to make progress with this issue, not only so that we can more confidently claim that our therapies work, but also so that we can start to tease apart which therapies work and why.

Part 3
Sentence processing

Chapter 3.1
Introduction

JANE MARSHALL

Language disordered children and adults may display particular problems in producing or understanding sentences. This may occur alongside lexical difficulties, or despite relative strengths with single words.

Problems with sentences manifest in a number of ways. For example, some individuals omit syntactic markers, such as function words and inflections:

> My er Mother died ... uh ... me ... uh ... fi'teen ... uh ... I guess six month ... my mother pass away ... and uh ... uh ... uh ... seventeen ... seventeen ... go uh High School (Badecker and Caramazza 1985)
> Mummy going the doctor's (Chiat unpublished)

Others have particular problems in composing word order:

> the man's running ... no ... the little girl's running in her arms ... her father's (target: a girl running into her father's arms; Saffran *et al.* 1980)

Still others make frequent verb errors, or omit verbs all together from their speech:

> the man is a sack of potatoes (target: carrying; McCarthy and Warrington 1985)
> I my flowers back (Rice and Bode 1993)

These different symptoms may co-occur. Indeed, some speakers produce little more than single nouns, with virtually no verbs, word order or syntactic markers:

> Mothers day ... er ... Nicola ... meals ... flowers ... er chocolates (Marshall *et al.* 1993)

Disordered sentence production is often accompanied by difficulties in sentence comprehension, although not always (e.g. Miceli *et al.* 1983,

Berndt 1987). Of course, many sentences, even syntactically complex ones, can be understood simply from the meaning of the content words. Take the following example:

The stallion with a bad hoof was ridden by the jockey in the red coat.

There is only one plausible relationship between the words in this sentence. Therefore, providing lexical comprehension is intact, it will be understood, even by someone with a severe grammatical impairment. This situation does not apply with semantically reversible sentences, such as

The jockey kicks the horse.

Here word order must be interpreted. As a result, reversible sentences often pose particular problems for people with a language disorder. In some cases, problems only appear with syntactically complex reversible sentences, while others fail with simple, subject verb object structures (Jones 1986, Schwartz *et al.* 1987, Van de Lely 1993).

It seems that sentence production and comprehension difficulties vary in both type and severity. One way of explaining these variations is to argue that they arise from different impairments in the sentence processing system. What might such a system look like?

Consider production first. One preliminary model has been offered by Garrett (e.g. 1988). This model contains a number of processing levels. The first is the **message level**, which determines the content of the message or idea to be communicated. Garrett sees this as a purely conceptual level. However, a number of other commentators (e.g. Levelt 1989, Pinker 1989) argue that, even here, processing is shaped by linguistic considerations. For example, when describing an event, the speaker must adopt a focus or perspective, and determine the main participants and their role. Furthermore, this information must be compatible with the verbs available to the speaker and their arguments. We can illustrate this in the context of the event shown in Figure 3.1.1. Here the speaker may focus on what is happening to the milk, the jug or even the bottle. These different perspectives influence the choice of verb and the eventual structure of the sentence, for example:

- The man pours the milk into the jug.
- The man fills the jug with milk.
- The man empties the bottle into the jug.

It seems that one basic requirement for talking about events is the ability to segment them into describable portions; and what is describable is largely determined by the contents of the speaker's verb lexicon.

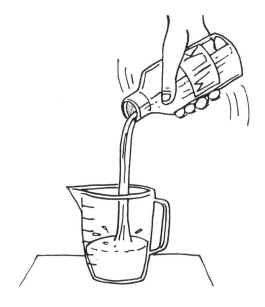

Figure 3.1 1

Garrett's next stage is called the **functional level**. Here a number of processes take place. First the speaker selects the main nouns and verbs. As already stated, these selections are influenced by earlier decisions about the event. Thus, in the examples above, a focus on the milk led to the selection of *pour* as the main verb, and *man*, *milk*, and *jug* as the key nouns. Secondly, the semantic relationship between the nouns and the verb is specified. This is partly determined by the semantic characteristics of the verb. *Pour* requires two arguments, or participants in the event. One participant performs the thematic role of **agent** (the person who initiates the action) and the other the role of **theme** (the thing that is moved by the action). It also permits an optional goal (or the destination of the transfer). The nouns are allocated to these role positions:

- agent = *man*
- theme = *milk*
- goal = *jug*

By now, the speaker has composed the semantic structure of the sentence (sometimes termed the **predicate argument structure**). Garrett argues that this representation is purely semantic. The speaker has no phonological information about the content words and has made no commitments to surface word order.

This processing is accomplished at the next level, the **positional level**. Here the phonological representations of the words are retrieved and the syntactic form selected. The latter might be envisaged as a grammatical frame, with gaps for the content word vocabulary, for example

the ... (N) ... is (V) + ing the ... (N) ... into the ... (N)

The phonological forms of the content words are slotted into these gaps. Now the speaker has a good idea of how the sentence will sound. The final stages in Garrett's model prepare the sentence for articulation.

Garrett's model has many advantages. In particular, it emphasises that not all sentence problems are related to syntax. Difficulties can also arise at the earlier semantic level, which specifies the meaning relations of the sentence, or in making the link between this level and the next. However, the model also leaves a number of processing questions unanswered, many of which bear upon these more semantic aspects of processing. For example, when composing the positional level representation, how does the speaker know where to place, or map, the content nouns, in order to convey the intended meaning? This is by no means a trivial problem. Indeed we encounter aphasic speakers who have difficulty precisely with this aspect of processing:

> in the ... pet shop, one woman and a cat is buying the man (target: a woman sells a cat to a man, from Marshall 1994)

Many people now agree (e.g. Levelt 1989, Haegeman 1991), that where to map the nouns in a sentence is largely dictated by the verb, at least when dealing with simple sentences. For example, *pour* tells us that the theme should be mapped on to the direct object position; whereas *fill* reserves direct object for the goal:

> pour the *milk* into the *jug* (theme *milk*, goal *jug*)
> fill the *jug* with *milk* (goal *jug*, theme *milk*)

These rules are not arbitrary but arise from the meaning of the verb. *Pour* describes the manner of movement, hence its affiliation with the theme, whereas *fill* describes the effect on the destination, hence its affiliation with the goal.

It seems that verb knowledge is crucial to production. The verb dictates the number of arguments involved in the event and where those arguments should be placed in the sentence. Furthermore, children seem able to exploit this type of verb information from a very early age. We know this from a number of experiments in which they are asked to learn novel verbs (see Pinker 1989). For example, they are shown an event in which a sponge is applied to some material to make it change colour. The child is told that this is *pilking*. Then a second event is demonstrated, in which the sponge is moved in a circuitous fashion until it comes to rest against the material. Now no colour change occurs. This event is described as *mooping*. Thus one of the novel verbs describes an event which affects the goal (*pilk*), whereas the other describes the manner of movement of the theme (*moop*). As a result, *pilk* should map the goal after the verb, while *moop* will map the theme after the verb. Interestingly, children as young as 3 seem sensitive to this rule. In other words, when asked to create sentences with these verbs they typically said: '*the man is pilking the cloth*' but '*the man is mooping the sponge*'.

These experiments show that children are able to extrapolate the structural properties of unfamiliar verbs purely from a demonstration of their meaning. We also know that children, from about 3 upwards, can exploit verb knowledge in the opposite direction; i.e. they can deduce the meaning of a novel verb largely from the structures in which it appears. In one experiment (Fisher *et al*. 1995), children were shown an event in which one toy animal chased another. Two descriptions of the event were offered; i.e some children heard 'the bunny is *zicking* the skunk' while the others heard 'the skunk is *blicking*'. Asked to explain the meaning of these verbs, the children correctly inferred that *zick* meant *chase* and *blick* meant *run away*. Given that they saw the same event, these inferences can only have been drawn from the structures used with the verbs.

It seems that children with normally developing language make automatic connections between the semantics and syntax of verbs; so much so, that they can infer the structural properties of verbs largely from their meaning, and the semantic properties largely from their syntax. Conversely, we can see that a verb impairment will have quite radical implications for the development of language. Not only would we anticipate impoverished verb production, we would also expect quite profound limitations in verb dependent structure. There is also a danger of a vicious circle being established, in that the inability to lay down verbs' semantic representations will impair the development of syntactic knowledge and this, in turn, will cut the child off from a potential route to verb meanings.

A number of studies have described semantic verb impairments in adults with aphasia (e.g. Jones 1986, Byng 1988, Mitchum and Berndt 1994). Although these subjects vary, they all display reduction in verb use and associated difficulties in composing and interpreting word order. Of course, unlike language-impaired children, these subjects once had a normal language system. As a result, we occasionally see quite striking dissociations. For example, subjects have been described who can still compose sophisticated syntactic structures, presumably by exploiting intact positional level skills, but cannot order the nouns in those structures in semantically appropriate ways (Martin and Blossom Stach 1986, Marshall 1994).

The insight that some sentence disorders in aphasia are due to semantic, rather than syntactic problems encouraged the development of semantic level therapies (e.g. Jones 1986, Byng 1988, Schwartz *et al.* 1994; see Marshall 1995 for review). These treatments, which are also termed **mapping therapy**, aim to give the individual better understanding of the underlying meaning relations of sentences, particularly by showing how those meanings are conveyed by the surface word order. Encouragingly, some positive results have been achieved by these interventions, both for production and comprehension. This encouraged the view that the semantic processing engaged by such treatments is common to both input and output.

Let us turn briefly to comprehension. As in production, comprehending sentences requires a number of processing elements or stages (see Black *et al.* 1992). The heard speech stream must be segmented into words and phrases, the syntactic structure of the sentence must be analysed and the meaning of the words accessed. Inferential processes are also brought to bear; i.e. the speaker interprets the meaning of the utterance against the developing discourse and his or her real world knowledge. The role of the verb is just as crucial in comprehension as it is in production. It defines the nature of the event and provides information about the possible arguments and their role. Thus when hearing the verb *pour* the listener knows that this is an event about liquid moving in a particular manner and that the noun phrase after the verb is almost certainly the theme.

An obvious question is whether sentence production and comprehension are accomplished by the same or separate systems. The similarity of processing might encourage the former view. For example, we might postulate one positional level, which computes syntactic forms in output and analyses the syntax of heard sentences in input. Although economical, this view is challenged by the evidence of dissociations in aphasia. For example, we encounter subjects whose comprehension of sentences is intact, but whose production is not (e.g. Miceli *et al.* 1983). Yet such dissociations may not call for entirely separate systems. It may be that impairments to a common module may have different implications for input and output, because of the different processing demands. We might also expect that elements of the systems may be shared, even if the whole system is not. In particular, as already suggested, it seems likely that both comprehension and production call upon the same semantic representations of verbs.

The following chapters describe a child and an adult with sentence level difficulties. There are a number of similarities between the cases. Both showed problems in dealing with verbs, and particularly the aspects of verbs which are critical in sentence processing. They are also given remarkably similar therapies. Yet the detail and consequences of their impairments, and their response to therapy, were quite different. These differences will be considered in the closing remarks. But first on to the cases.

Chapter 3.2
Colourful semantics: thematic role therapy

ALISON BRYAN

How often have you read an article or listened to a case study and found yourself recognising the picture of the client being described? Your interest in the assessment and therapy procedures is then coloured with enthusiastic thoughts of their application to a member of your own case load. It is likely that there is some basic common ground, such as the fact that they are both children! However, what do you do when the description you've read is of a stroke patient and your client is a 5 year old with a specific speech and language disorder? This is what happened to me when I read Eirian Jones's (1986) case study of BB.

BB was a 41 year old who suffered a left CVA leaving him with a Broca's type aphasia. At the time of the study he had a severe word finding deficit and his output was predominant single nouns with no sentence structures. He also had a severe sentence comprehension deficit, which particularly impaired his understanding of reversible sentences. Despite these difficulties BB had some syntactic skills. For example, he could readily identify the syntactic phrases within written sentences. Jones therefore hypothesised that his problems were more semantic, at the level of creating the predicate argument structure. This hypothesis was derived from the application of the normal sentence processing model put forward by Garrett (1980).

During her investigations with BB, Jones (1986) observed that he was very preoccupied with positional level elements of the sentence, such as function words and inflections, and became very concerned if he could not access these features. She hypothesised that this reflected previous therapy regimes which had emphasised correct surface structure.

It was this observation that first struck a chord. When I gave my client, Gordon, a picture description task, he tended to over-emphasise the function words. He frequently started with a heavily stressed and inflected '*the*' followed by a pause while he searched for the subject lexical item. A similar over-emphasis then occurred on the auxiliary '*is*' before accessing the stem of the verb. It is interesting to note that

Gordon's previous language programme was aimed at improving the phrase structure (positional level) of SVO type sentences.

Subject information

At the time of the study Gordon was 5 years 10 months and had been in an infant speech and language unit for 5 months.

His birth history was unremarkable and all developmental mile-stones, apart from speech and language, were achieved in the normal range (e.g. walked at 11 months). Gordon had no history of hearing impairment, passing all the developmental tests. He had no major illnesses other than the usual childhood infections.

Gordon came from a very supportive two-parent family and had an older sister whose speech and language development was normal. Gordon's mother reported that she herself didn't speak until she was about 2.06 to 3, but had no subsequent difficulties. There was no other family history of speech and language or hearing problems.

Gordon's first word was reported at the age of 2 years but there was little development after this, with Gordon relying on pointing and gesture plus a few non-specific vocalisations to communicate.

Gordon was referred to the speech and language therapy service at the age of 2 years 7 months. At this time he still only had 3–4 recognis-able words. His comprehension, social skills and listening and attention skills were reported to be within normal limits. Initially his play skills were reported to be mildly delayed.

Gordon became extremely anxious whenever his communication skills were the focus of attention. After the initial few appointments it became obvious that direct 1:1 intervention would not be possible at that time. Gordon attended various language development and listening/discrimination groups from the age of 2 years 11 months to 4 years 5 months.

By this time Gordon was still very wary of 1:1 intervention, although in the groups he would now attempt some sound and word imitation. He had acquired more single words but was still relying on supporting these with gesture, symbolic noise and isolated sounds (e.g. /k/ for *car*).

A statement of special educational needs was initiated and at 4 years 5 months Gordon entered a pre-school unit which served both hearing impaired and speech and language disordered children. Initially all intervention was aimed at boosting his self-confidence and gradually he began to cope with direct intervention in his weekly therapy sessions. Makaton signing was taught and its use encouraged. Language develop-ment was targeted at expanding the number of word combinations. He worked on sound imitation and sound sequencing skills plus oral motor exercises.

At 5 years 5 months Gordon was transferred to the infant speech and language unit. He now had a wide variety of single words and was using some 3–4 word phrases although there was evidence of both word retrieval, particularly at sentence planning level, and word order difficulties. His oral motor skills were significantly better. His phonology was delayed, showing blend reduction, occasional stopping and de-affrication of affricates. His articulation and imitation skills were significantly improved, but he still had a few vowel distortions (e.g. *clown* – /klæn /) and some syllable reduction (e.g. *elephant* – / efənt /). Gordon was generally intelligible in single words but his intelligibility was sometimes reduced when he was having planning problems at the sentence level.

Gordon's comprehension was tested on the Reynell Developmental Language Scales (Reynell and Huntly 1985). This is a toy-based test in which the child has to select or move miniature toys according to spoken instructions of increasing complexity of structure and vocabulary. At chronological age 5 years 7 months his standard score was –0.7, which was just about within normal limits.

Investigations

I first met Gordon in his second term at the speech and language therapy unit (chronological age 5 years 10 months). The most striking thing about his expressive language skills at this time was their great variability. Apart from familiar social phrases, his best utterances were connected with simple picture description activities. However, in settings where there was no pictorial support Gordon's utterances were significantly shorter, with greater word retrieval and word order problems. The worst scenario for him was always the weekly 'news' session where the children had to relate their weekend's activities to the rest of the class. In this situation Gordon was frequently reduced to an anxious silence and eventually a single word after much prompting. He just didn't seem to be able to get started. His previous therapist reported that a major concern was Gordon's inability to generalise the sentence construction skills evident in therapy activities.

One of Gordon's strengths was his literacy skills. His reading was age appropriate in that he could recognise a variety of words using the logographic (whole word) approach together with context clues and initial letter recognition to attempt unfamiliar vocabulary. He had a core of words from the Breakthrough Scheme (Mackay and Thompson 1970) which he could write from memory. He could also easily copy write or write to dictation any word he didn't know. Application of his written language skills was severely restricted by his expressive language problems. He could create a sentence aloud with a lot of support but was unable to hold on to that sentence long enough to write it down.

As part of Gordon's general assessment two standardised tests for expressive language skills had already been administered (Renfrew's Bus Story and Action Picture Test). Further examples of output were collected from informal picture description tasks, spontaneous utterances and Gordon's efforts in 'news time'.

Standardised tests

Two tests were administered (see Table 3.2.1). In the Bus Story, Gordon was told a narrative about a runaway bus, which he had to re-tell with the support of pictures. The Renfrew Action Picture Test is a simple

Table 3.2.1 Pre-therapy samples and scores from the Bus Story and Action Picture Test

Bus Story (chronological age 5 years 8 months)
T: *Once upon a*
G: time ...
T: *What's this?*
G: bus
T: *And what happened?*
G: ...one other man
T: *What did the bus do?*
G: run ... train ... race a bus ... mmmm ...
T: *What happened here?*
G: ...train ... er ...
T: *Where's the train gone?*
G: train in ...
T: *In a tu ...?*
G: tunnel ... nother place ... man whistle here ... stop ...
T: *Did he stop?*
G: mmm ...yea ... jump over fence ... talking cow here ... race down in water here ... put on brakes here? man in bus now

Information = 7, below mean for chronological age 3 years
Average 5 longest sentences = 3.5, below mean for chronological 3 years

Action Picture Test (chronological age 5 years 10 months)
1. the girl skipping
2. cuddling a ... teddy bear
3. on the head ... bowl ... on the head
4. the ... girl jumper over ... a gate
5. the ... cat ... catch a mouse
6. fall down the steps ... broken the glasses
7. 'kow' baby up the post office (target a woman holds a child who is posting a letter)
8. riding up the ladder ... get the cat
9. girl 'puttit' flowers in the ...

Information = 20, mean for chronological age 4 years 6 months
Grammar = 14, below mean for chronological age 3 years

picture description task. Gordon needed a great deal of prompting and support with leading questions to complete the Bus Story (see the therapists prompts in Table 3.2.1). This was taken into account when scoring and some prompted utterances were not counted.

Non-standardised picture descriptions

Gordon was asked to describe the What's Wrong cards (LDA Materials) and some story sequence cards. Examples of his responses are shown in Table 3.2.2.

Table 3.2.2 Pre-therapy examples of picture description

Best responses
tree have shoes
duck have ride in a boat
lady have banana on head
the bike have square wheels
slide come apart

Verb problems	**target**
dog up a ... run up a sky	a dog walking in the sky
man have carrot on hand	holding
lady upside down pencil	holding/using

Other problems	
kettle ... um ... teeshirt	a woman ironing with a kettle
sausages have breakfast	pouring sausages out of a cereal packet
open window mummy	a woman opening a window
hanger in the ...	clothes hanging in the cooker
the dog is have ... dog ... have dog's	a boy pouring biscuits into the dog's bowl
biscuits ... and then have eat them	and the dog eats them

The following trends emerged in Gordon's picture descriptions.

1. There were significant difficulties with lexical retrieval, especially with verbs. This is shown in:

    - an over-reliance on the non-specific verb *have*
    - the omission of verbs, e.g. 'lady upside down pencil'
    - the use of neologistic verbs, some of which may have been a blend of two targets, e.g. 'kow baby up the post office'
    - the presence of semantic errors, e.g. 'post office' for *post box* and 'ride up' for *climb*

2. There was an over reliance on SVO sentences, even when this structure was inappropriate, e.g. 'sausages have breakfast'

3. There were occasional word order problems, e.g. 'open window mummy'
4. Some utterances were executed very slowly with several pauses in between clause elements, e.g. 'the cat ... catch ... the mouse'.

Spontaneous utterances

Gordon's difficulties were even more marked in unstructured situations. Some typical examples are given in Table 3.2.3, which show word order problems, omission of clause elements and a dependence on single word utterances. There were also frequent periods of long silences when he was put on the spot. It was evident from his facial expressions that he was trying to respond but was unable to do so.

Table 3.2.3 Pre-therapy examples of spontaneous utterances

	Possible target
news me like	I like the news
out now?	Can I go out now?
tissue	I need a tissue
... Burger King	I went to Burger King
um ... um ... book bag	I put it in my book bag (in answer to 'where did you put your speech therapy book?')

Comprehension

Although Gordon's comprehension was adequate on the standardised test, I also informally investigated his comprehension of verbs and reversible sentences. In one task, he had to match a spoken verb to one of four semantically related verb pictures. This caused him no problems. In another task, he heard a sentence which had to be matched to one of two pictures (the target and its reversal). He was also asked to judge whether a spoken sentence matched a presented picture. These tasks included pragmatically anomalous sentences, such as 'the banana ate the girl'. Gordon had no difficulties with the sentence level tasks. His ability to cope with the highly unlikely sentences showed that he could interpret word order correctly, even when the meaning flouted pragmatic expectations.

Conclusions from the investigations

It is obvious from these examples that Gordon has significant problems with sentence construction and word retrieval, especially when there is no picture support. I have already mentioned that the initial impression of over-emphasis on function words led me to see a similarity between

Gordon and BB (Jones 1986). If we now re-examine these examples with reference to the functional level of the Garrett model, further similarities emerge:

- **Lexical selection** Like BB, Gordon had problems accessing both verbs and nouns.
- **Creation of a predicate argument structure** A problem with creating the underlying predicate argument structure could account for many of the sentence construction difficulties seen here. Like BB, Gordon was frequently reduced to using single words.

Unlike BB, Gordon could create short sentences, some of which combined up to two arguments with a verb. We also see some variability in the range of semantic relations conveyed. For example, Gordon expresses agent/patient relations (as in 'cat ... catch the mouse'), location ('man in bus now') and possession ('lady have banana on head').

However, Gordon's skills seemed heavily dependent on the nature of the stimulus. His best output was achieved in simple picture description, or when he had been cued by a previously heard narrative, as in the Bus Story. His production was much more vulnerable in spontaneous speech, or when he had to make inferences from the pictures, as was often the case with the What's Wrong cards. In these conditions, a number of problems emerged. Many of Gordon's utterances lacked a verb, or were built around inappropriate verbs. Even when a verb was achieved, Gordon often had difficulty creating an appropriate structure. This resulted in word order errors, such as 'open window mummy' and 'news I like'; the omission of arguments which were essential to the message, such as 'talking cow here' or totally anomalous output, such as 'sausages have breakfast'.

Gordon seemed to have particular problems describing multiple events, in which several arguments are involved and in which more than one action is taking place. Here, he tended to omit one element, e.g. 'Kow baby up the post office' (target: a woman holds up a child who is posting a letter). When he attempted all elements his output tended to break down, e.g.: 'the dog is have ... dog ... have dog's biscuits ... and then have eat them' (a boy pours biscuits into the dog's bowl and the dog eats them).

In Jones's study, investigations showed that BB could retrieve verbs in isolation but seemed to have no knowledge of how to use the verb and its arguments to mark underlying meaning relations. We have seen that Gordon can sometimes create the predicate argument structure particularly when there is picture support, although at times this is still inappropriate for the intended meaning. In less structured contexts Gordon's problems are magnified. When he can come up with some structure it is often anomalous or incomplete.

It was therefore decided to adapt the therapy regime Jones used with BB to try to raise Gordon's awareness of the predicate argument structure of sentences to a conscious level. With BB, the therapy consisted of **input** activities which aimed to illuminate the connections between the surface form of a sentence and the underlying meaning relations. However Gordon's problem seemed to be at least partially one of using the knowledge he had and also needing to extend the variety of structures. Thus with Gordon it was felt appropriate also to include an **output** component in the therapy. It was hoped that by keeping the focus very much on the functional level Gordon would not be concerned about the phrase structure elements.

Therapy

The rationale behind Gordon's therapy programme was that by focusing on the functional rather than positional level, Gordon would become more aware of the underlying predicate argument structure of sentences. I hypothesised that this would, in turn, encourage him to use and extend his skills in creating predicate argument structure during output. The therapy would be carried out initially through the analysis and construction of written sentences. If the hypothesis that this targets the true level of his difficulties is correct we should see carryover of therapy benefits into everyday communication. The true test therefore of this therapy regime would be an improvement in his spontaneous offerings at 'news time'.

The aims of the therapy were twofold.

* To teach the identification of underlying thematic roles in written sentences.
* To encourage the use of thematic role knowledge to create the following predicate argument structures in written sentences:
     verb: agent, theme
     verb: agent, location
     verb: agent, theme, location
     verb: theme, description.

Following the therapy regime for BB, it was decided that each thematic role would be identified by and linked with a question form. This would be both said and signed (Paget–Gorman Sign System). In addition each thematic role and associated question was assigned a colour code. This was used in several ways:

* to discriminate visually between each thematic role
* to further establish the relationship between the question and the thematic role

- to associate each target sentence type with a visual colour sequence
- to cue Gordon when he omitted a thematic role

Gordon had not been taught Paget–Gorman formally. It was used periodically in the unit to sign key words, especially concepts. He was, however, used to signs, since he had been taught a basic Makaton vocabulary in clinic and in the pre-school unit to support his expressive attempts.

Colour coding of sentence construction is not a new concept in working with language disordered children. For example, the Language Through Reading scheme (1981) which is based on the LARSP (Crystal *et al*. 1982), uses colour coding. In this scheme phrase structure elements are colour coded, e.g. nouns are orange, verbs are yellow and determiners are white. This is a coding of the surface grammar of the sentence, or the **positional level** if we refer to Garrett's model. Although this scheme was used in Gordon's speech and language unit, the colour coding element was not. The colour coding in Gordon's therapy was different. Here, in association with the question forms, Gordon was asked to segment written sentences into their thematic roles and colour code these. Thus the colour coding reflected the predicate argument structure (**functional level**) of the sentence. The colour coding system is given in Table 3.2.4.

Table 3.2.4 The colour coding system used in Gordon's therapy

Question	Colour coding	Referent
What doing	yellow	verb
Who	orange	agent
What	green	theme
Where	red	location
What like	blue	description

Gordon was seen individually four times a week for 20–30 minutes. He also took home colour coding activities at least once a week. After the first week the colour coding was also introduced into his news writing session.

The therapy programme

Step 1

Gordon was presented with simple SV pictures and colour coded sentences cut up into the two elements of **agent** (orange) and **verb** (yellow). The first SV pictures from the LTR (Language Through Reading scheme) were used and the cut up sentences were either on coloured card or on white card but written in the appropriate colour (see Figure 3.2.1).

The lady (orange)	*is walking* (yellow)

Figure 3.2.1 Colour coded sentence elements

The therapist signed and asked '**Who** is it?'and Gordon had to find the **agent**. The colour link was then established by saying 'yes, that's **who**. **Who** words are orange'.

Next the therapist signed and asked 'What's she **doing**?' and Gordon had to find the **verb**. The colour link was then established by the therapist saying 'yes, that's what she is **doing**. The **doing** words are yellow'. Gordon then had to put the cards in the right order. He had no problems with this and the process was repeated with a variety of sentences, all with animate actors and present progressive tense verbs.

Next, the same sentences were presented as a whole, with the pictures, and Gordon had to underline the **agent** and the **verb** in the appropriate colours. Each time the question word and colour link was emphasised. Gordon had no problems with underlining all the surface phrase elements that go together to make up each thematic role. Like BB he instinctively knew where each thematic role started and finished. Finally a variety of similar sentences were presented without pictures and Gordon colour coded these.

Step 2

The role of theme was introduced in the same way. Sentences were presented (with and without pictures) which were cut up into the three elements of **agent**, **verb** and **theme**. The theme role was identified using the question word and sign for **what**. The colour link was established by the therapist's feedback. For example, I might say: 'yes, that's **what** he's eating. **What** words are green'. By now, it was not always necessary to have a picture with the sentence when reconstructing it.

Unlike BB, Gordon had no difficulty in re-ordering the cards to give the correct structure. This was further evidence that Gordon had some knowledge of how to map underlying meaning relations, but had difficulty applying this knowledge in his spoken and written output. As before, Gordon was now given a variety of uncoded written sentences and asked to underline the verb and two thematic roles. We introduced a wider variety of verb vocabulary in various tenses, but kept the agent animate and the theme inanimate.

Additional therapy tasks were now given to reinforce the links between the thematic role, the question word and the colour. These can be seen in Figure 3.2.2. In tasks where Gordon had to create his own

1. Re-assembling sentences cut up into their thematic roles and individually colour coded

is eating (yellow)	Gordon (orange)
in the kitchen (red)	chips (green)

2. Underlining, in the appropriate colour, all the words that go with each thematic role in written sentences

3. Writing sentences describing pictures on a colour coded sentence pattern. [i.e. an orange line, then yellow line, then green line]

4. Underlining a target role in several sentences
   e.g. 'Underline all the **doing** words in **yellow**'

4. Filling in missing roles in sentences describing SVO pictures
   e.g. _ _ _ _ _ is at school   [_ _ _ _ _ =orange]
   She..........................a horse   [.......... = yellow]
   He ate his_____   [_____= green]

5. Answering colour coded questions by writing on a colour coded sentence pattern
   e.g. 'At snack time **what** do you eat?'

   _ _ _ _ _:....................._____

6. The child asks the therapist the cue questions related to written sentences using the signs. The therapist then has to answer the question and colour code the correct thematic role.

7. The child dictates a sentence and the therapist writes down the appropriate coloured lines. The child then 'reads back' the sentence following the lines. He/she can then write it down on the lines. This was used particularly in writing Gordon's weekly 'news'.

8. The child is cued when he/she omits a thematic role in conversation
   i.e. 'I didn't hear **who**/the orange word'

Figure 3.2.2 Therapy tasks.

sentences, he occasionally had difficulty retrieving the verb. It was essential to establish the correct verb before carrying on in case of incompatibility of the possible argument structures.

At this stage, it was also sometimes possible to cue Gordon into using the verbs and thematic roles he had omitted in conversation. For example, he wanted me to write some homework in his book and said 'in my book'. I told him that he had forgotten the 'who' and the 'doing' words. I then wrote down what he had said but put an orange and yellow line before it. When asked to try again using the coded lines he said 'You write in my book please'.

Step 3

The thematic role of **location** was introduced in the same way. This was coloured red and cued with the question '**where?**'. Gordon very quickly integrated this into a variety of tasks. He had no problem discriminating between sentences taking a theme mapped on to a direct object and sentences taking a location, mapped on to a prepositional phrase, and colour coded them appropriately. At this stage copulas were introduced in the verb role (e.g. Gordon **is at** school). Gordon did not have a problem recognising these as 'doing' words. Ideally they should perhaps have been called 'being' words but I thought this would have added unnecessary confusion.

Step 4

Tasks now employed sentences with a verb and all three thematic roles, i.e. by using structures with both a direct object and prepositional phrase after the verb. Gordon initially needed help to find all three roles, since he tended to underline the theme and location together in answer to the question '**what**'. He had no problems in the other tasks which involved re-assembly or filling in missing spaces.

Step 5

Gordon was then introduced to inanimate objects in the **agent** role. This initially caused a problem, since they do not answer the question '**who**'. This was eventually overcome by emphasising the colour coding aspect, i.e. 'These are also orange words'. I also encouraged the use of more pronouns in the agent role (I, he, she, it). Gordon frequently omitted the agent role in conversation when use of a subject pronoun was appropriate.

Interim reevaluation

At this point Gordon had been following the therapy programme for about 4–5 weeks. Already an improvement in his spontaneous output was being commented on by staff and his parents. He was using more sentences containing a verb and two, and occasionally three, thematic roles. If he omitted a role he could often be cued with the question word or colour. There were still times when he could not begin a response but these were less frequent. Examples of his spoken and written 'news' at this time can be seen in Table 3.2.5. It was decided to continue the therapy programme.

Table 3.2.5 Examples of spontaneous news (spoken and written) during and after therapy

4–5 weeks into the programme
I played with my friend at his house (spoken)
I watched tele (spoken)

8 weeks into the programme
I have my Easter egg (at) home (written, bracketed item indicates adult correction)
I see Hook ... Hook is a baddie ... I see the pirate ship ... my tooth hurts (spoken)
I stayed at home ... watched tele all day long (spoken)

3 months after the start of the programme
my sister go to my carnival on Sunday .. my nanny coming over on Sunday have dinner in the dining room ... Claire holding the bucket ... money in it ... my nanny go home on Sunday ... at night (spoken)

Step 6

We continued with reinforcement of all the thematic roles introduced so far using similar therapy tasks (see Figure 3.2.2). Meanwhile we introduced a role to represent a complement (I've called it **description**), in answer to the question 'What is it like?'. This was colour coded blue.

Initially there was some confusion between the underlying roles in SV and SVComplement sentences, because of their similar surface structures, e.g.

'she is eating'	vs	'she is tall'
(agent, verb)		**(theme, verb, description)**

Gordon tended to mark the description word as part of the verb. This was soon resolved by asking the '**what doing**' question about both words he had coloured yellow. He could then sort out that *tall* was not a doing word but marked '**What's it like**'.

Step 7

By this time Gordon was using more than one sentence for his news and when describing picture sequences. He tended to omit the agent in all but the first sentence. We therefore worked on reiteration of the agent in written sentence sequences, using pronouns where appropriate. He also never coordinated any of the sentences so, although it is not an element of predicate argument structure (nor is verb or description a thematic role), we chose '**and**' to be our linking word in purple.

Further reevaluation

We had now been running the programme for about 8 weeks. Gordon's spontaneous language showed striking improvements. He was using several short sentences in 'news time' (see Table 3.2.5) and was much more confident when put on the spot for an answer or comment. He was still quite hesitant in his planning at times, and his word retrieval problems were now very much in evidence as he attempted to use more complete sentences. He would have to pause and search for a word or use a semantically related alternative. If he was unsuccessful, then he would just trail off and sometimes try again using a different sentence structure. If it was evident from the context what the target was, sometimes the adult would supply the word or give a phonic cue to enable Gordon to complete the sentence. Gordon seemed to have equal difficulty retrieving verbs and nouns although this was not objectively measured.

It is interesting to note that, at this point, I had only one instance of any word order errors either in picture description or in spontaneous utterances. Gordon was able to correct this when it was pointed out.

It was decided to continue using the colour coding as a basis for some of his written work and as a strategy for correction. At this time it was felt that Gordon was still gaining benefit from generalising his new sentence construction skills at this level, so no new colour coding was introduced. We were also interested in whether his sentence construction skills could develop further without direct intervention. So, for the next half term individual therapy focused on improving his lexical retrieval skills, particularly for verbs. Given the semantic focus of the tasks, this therapy was still pitched at the **functional level** of processing. Therapy tasks focused on:

- **verb–noun** links; e.g. naming object functions, thinking of three objects to go with one verb. (He found this work hard, especially when he had to find more than one association.)
- teaching **target verbs** with sign support
- **description of objects** by associate features
- **semantic circles** (i.e. generating or judging **noun–noun** associations)
- teaching **strategies** to signal word retrieval problems, e.g. '*I've forgotten*'.

Colour coding was used when necessary to support Gordon's incidental sentence construction. We also worked on some phonological awareness skills and articulation of *sh* and *ch*.

Outcome

Improvements at the functional level

Table 3.2.5 shows that there was a marked improvement in Gordon's spontaneous speech during the first 8 weeks of the programme, while Gordon was being taught to identify and use thematic roles through colour coding. This improvement continued over the next half term, when therapy was used to support, rather than teach, sentence construction. In the 3 months from initiating this programme Gordon's 'news' went from being occasional words to four or five sentences, consisting of a verb combined with up to three argument and non-argument phrases, although he still had problems with lexical retrieval and the flow of his sentences could still be quite hesitant as he struggled to plan them.

In addition both the pre-therapy standardised tests were administered. The transcripts and scores can be seen in Table 3.2.6. Gordon's information scores greatly improved in both standardised tests. In the 5 months between testing, his information score on the Action Picture Test progressed by 12–18 months. In the 7 months between testing in the Bus Story, Gordon's information score advanced by 12 months. This could just mean that he was able to retrieve more vocabulary, but if we look at the transcript we can see the majority of the sentences have the correct predicate argument structure. We also see an improvement in his ability to describe complex events, in which more than one action is taking place (e.g. no. 7 in the Action Picture Test). Although the average of the five longest sentences on the Bus Story is still below the scale, it has gone up from 3.5 words to 6 words, indicating more complex sentence structures.

Table 3.2.7 looks more closely at the number of verbs and verb argument structures produced by Gordon in these tests, before and after therapy (the analysis excludes false starts and heavily cued utterances). This table shows a number of gains. First, Gordon clearly uses more verbs after therapy. Before therapy the samples contain 18 verbs (10 in the Action Picture Test and 8 in the bus story). After therapy the number increases to 33 (18 in the Action Picture Test and 15 in the Bus Story). Furthermore, only 2 of these post-therapy verbs could be classed as errors. Secondly the analysis shows a striking increase in the number of utterances containing verb argument structure. In particular, there are many more utterances which combine two arguments with a verb after therapy.

So, we can see a dramatic improvement in Gordon's ability to create appropriate verb argument structures, as evidenced both in improved standardised information scores and in his ability to tell his 'news'. Furthermore, these gains happened over a relatively short period of time. The results would seem to support the original therapy hypothesis that

Table 3.2.6 Post-therapy samples and scores from the Bus Story and Action Picture Tests

---

Bus Story (chronological age 6 years 3 months)

T: *Once upon a time*
G: the bus ... um ... um ... and he fixing the bus
   and ... bus run away
   the ... bus met the train
   the train going under the tunnel
   and he is alone
   and he go in the town
   and he blow the whistle ...'stop'
   the bus run away again
   the man ... the bus jump over the gate
   met the cow in the field
   and the bus run ... falling down the ... um ... hill
   and fall in the water
   and the bus ... um... hook them the lorry
   get on the road again

	pre-therapy	**post-therapy**
Information	7 (< mean for CA 3;00)	22 (mean for CA 4;0)
Average 5 longest sentences	3.5 (< mean for CA 3;00)	6 (< mean for CA 3;0)

Action Picture Test (chronological age 6 years 3 months)
1. she holding the teddy
2. he ... putting ... she um ... putting he ... she boots on
3. the dog ... um ... the dog ... um ... holding the ... the ... on the wood
4. the man jumping over the gate
5. the cat ... um ... getting the mouse
6. the ... um ... she ... falling down the stairs ... broken the glasses ... she crying
7. she um ... lifting the baby up ... put the letter in ... in the post office
8. he climb up the ladder ... get the cat
9. he ... she ... he ... the dog taking the shoe off he foot
10. the lady dropping ... got hole on it ... in the bag ... the apples falling out and she haven't got the apples ... he picking the apples up

	pre-therapy	**post-therapy**
Information Score	20 (CA 4;06)	31 (CA 5;06–5;11)
Grammar	14 (< mean for CA 3;0)	8.5 (< mean for CA 3;6) (revised edition)

Gordon's difficulties were in creating an appropriate predicate argument structure at the functional level of sentence processing in unstructured settings. His therapy regime was targeted at teaching awareness of the relationships between the thematic roles that make up this structure. By linking the thematic roles with question words their relationship to the verb was emphasised. Colour coding the roles further emphasised the relationships between them, at least in simple active sentences.

Table 3.2.7 Pre-and post-therapy analysis of the verb argument structures used by Gordon in the Bus Story and Action Picture Tests

Utterance type	No. of utterances produced	
	pre-therapy	post-therapy
Verb alone	2	1
Single noun phrase	5	0
Conjoined phrases without a verb	2	0
Verb + 1 argument	10	6
Verb + 2 arguments	5*	23
Verb + 3 arguments	0	1
Verb + 1 argument + 1 non- argument phrase	1	2

*in one utterance the verb was realised as a neologism 'kow'.

Positional level

It is interesting to note that, after therapy, some positional level elements were being used correctly in unstructured settings, despite not being targeted. For example, Gordon's utterances contained more determiners, occasional copulas, and past tense forms. Some negative structures also appeared, which were well beyond the scope of the therapy programme. For example, he said 'I haven't got my coat' which previously would have come out as 'Got my coat no'.

An analysis of some positional level information from the pre-and post-therapy tests can be seen in table 3.2.8. This shows an improvement in his use of pronouns and the coordinator 'and'. Both of these were highlighted during the therapy programme. However there is also a striking increase in the complexity of verb tense marking and a decrease in idiosyncratic verb marking. These were not specifically highlighted in therapy, although a variety of verb markers were used in the tasks. These gains may have come about for two reasons. Gordon's improved semantic skills may have activated improved processing at the positional level. Alternatively, this processing might always have been available. However, prior to therapy Gordon might have been unable to use it, because of his difficulties at the earlier, functional level.

A similar picture of improvement was seen in Gordon's written work. By the end of the programme Gordon could decide on simple sentences he wanted to write and could retain them in his head while writing them down, without any colour coding lines. It was interesting to note that although he sometimes omitted positional level information, he could often supply this information if the sentence was read aloud to him.

Table 3.2.8 Positional level information in the Bus Story and Action Picture samples

	Pre-therapy	Post-therapy
Number of pronouns produced	0	16
Number of uses of coordinator *and*	0	7
Verb markers used (% of total)		
Stem alone	59	41
Inflected	29	50
Irregular whole word past forms	0	3
Copular	0	3
Plus auxiliary	0	3
Idiosyncratic verb forms	12	0

It is suggested that the improvement seen in Gordon's spontaneous spoken sentence structure is due to therapy being correctly aimed at the functional level. This contrasts with the lack of carryover when therapy was targeted at the positional level. The speed with which Gordon progressed seems to confirm the impression that, unlike BB, he already had underlying knowledge of predicate argument structure but was unable to apply it. Possibly, therapy enabled him to access, use and build on this knowledge at a conscious level in less structured settings.

There are obvious implications of the success of this therapy regime for other language disordered children. If therapy is to be effective it is vital that it is targeted at the correct level(s) of processing. Although Gordon did have positional level errors, the main source of his difficulties was at the functional level. Tools such as the Language, Assessment, Remediation and Screening Procedure (Crystal *et al*. 1982) can profile the range of syntactic structures used by a child, but do not profile the range of meaning relations expressed. It is therefore vital to analyse at the deeper functional level, particularly looking at utterances with errors in word order, thematic role selection and lexical retrieval.

It should be said that not all children will have Gordon's literacy skills, but this doesn't preclude thematic role therapy. Use of schemes such as levels 2–4 of the Derbyshire Language Scheme help both therapist and child to keep focused on the underlying thematic roles involved in understanding and creating sentences. In addition I have used Makaton symbols instead of written words to create sentences on colour coded lines.

Gordon's comprehension abilities were such that he could cope well with all elements of the therapy. Other children might well have difficulties understanding the question words. In their case, signing question words and using colour coding could be helpful. Some children may have difficulties understanding or creating reversible sentences (e.g. *The boy hit the girl*). Here again the question words and colour coding could help to sort out the underlying meaning relationships.

Finally, as with BB, this therapy could be extended to far more complex sentences. I have used thematic role coding to demonstrate the relationship between the surface word order and the underlying meaning relations in passive voice sentences.

As therapists, we know that there are rarely any completely new therapy tasks. It is the application of these tasks that changes. We have all used question words to elicit elements of sentences in picture description. The difference with thematic role therapy is that this coding aims to illuminate the relationship between the questions and the underlying meaning relationships of the sentence. If successful, the child will hopefully use this knowledge, without the therapist having to be there to ask the questions!

Chapter 3.3
Mapping therapy with a fluent dysphasic?

SUSAN PETHERS

In the last decade there have been several studies describing 'mapping therapies' with aphasic individuals (e.g. Jones 1986, Byng 1988). Rather than focusing on syntax, these therapies aimed to remediate the semantic aspects of sentence production and comprehension, particularly by illuminating the connections between the surface word order of a sentence and the underlying meaning relations. A recent development suggested that, for some individuals, additional work at the level of event processing might be incorporated into mapping programmes (Marshall *et al.* 1993).

Mapping problems are usually linked with an agrammatic presentation. The subject described in this paper is different, in that he had a fluent dysphasia. However, he also presented with some classic 'mapping symptoms', such as poor sentence comprehension and production, verb errors and the reversal of arguments. This suggested that mapping therapy should be considered.

Background

PT is a husband, the father of two teenage daughters, and a former assistant bank manager. One Saturday in August 1993, when he was 39, he played an early round of golf, returned home and collapsed in the bathroom.

Neurological information and recovery

A CT scan revealed a massive infarction in left middle cerebral artery territory affecting posterior frontal, temporal and temporoparietal regions. The CVA was probably related to a blood disorder, undetected until the event, and resulted in a right sided hemiparesis (weakness) and severe expressive and receptive dysphasia. The CVA was so severe that the family were informed he was unlikely to survive.

However, 1 month later PT transferred to the rehabilitation unit. The hemiparesis had improved, and he was independently mobile, though requiring supervision for all daily living activities. Some cognitive difficulties were noted at this time. These included reduced short term memory, reduced speed of processing and problem solving skills, together with perseverative and rigid thinking. He also appeared very inhibited and lacking in confidence.

By report, PT was usually silent, producing occasional social greetings and the odd appropriate single word. When pushed to converse he produced fluent jargon. Functional comprehension was very poor, and he seemed unable to use non-verbal cues to support his language. PT described this experience immediately post-CVA as the most frightening and bewildering time of his life. He returned home from the rehabilitation unit in January 1994 at 5 months post-onset. Since discharge, PT has been neurologically stable, apart from two brief fits, one at 7 and the other at 25 months post-onset. These had caused no apparent residual effects.

Social and family information

PT left school after 'A' levels having been offered a post in a bank, and stayed there throughout his career, working his way up. He met his wife LT at school, and they married in their early twenties. LT describes her husband pre-CVA as quiet, shy and meticulous. He worked extremely long hours and brought work home in the evenings. At the weekend he played golf with a close friend, or went to the occasional football or cricket match.

Following the CVA, PT had to retire from the bank. He took up wood working, and made planters, carved cupboards and so on for family and friends. Although his wife and daughters are artistic, PT had not previously considered himself to be creative. PT reported that he did not miss the bank. However, he did seem to value himself less since he was not able to carry out those tasks which he formerly did so well. After his stroke, PT's social contacts were mainly with his immediate family, his parents and his grandfather. Otherwise, he preferred working alone to meeting people.

Former therapy

Assessment of PT's language when he entered the rehabilitation unit suggested a central semantic impairment. This manifested even in non-verbal tasks. For example he scored just 38/52 on the Pyramids and Palm Trees Test, in which he had to match pictures on the basis of a semantic association. It also affected the comprehension and production of single words. When asked to match spoken words to pictures he scored only

25/40, all his errors involving the selection of semantically related items (Psycholinguistic Assessment of Language Processing in Aphasia, PALPA; Kay *et al.* 1992). He was unable to produce the spoken names of pictures, although he did marginally better in writing (6/16). Sentence comprehension, as measured on the TROG (Test for Reception of Grammar, Bishop 1982), was impossible. His connected speech was virtually uninterpretable, as this example shows:

> Two martin bits with this thing here ... she's reading that one there ... she's the pins that one's by the thing there ... that one's its um is a ... its a ... making it faster ... its that fising that bit there ... (Description of the Cookie Theft Picture, Boston Diagnostic Aphasia Examination)

Early therapy focused on strengthening semantic accessing for nouns, then verbs. This involved input tasks, such as synonym judgements, and output tasks such as production of associates. Drawing was also encouraged for output, and during therapy PT's pictures became increasingly neat, precise and detailed, suggesting increasing semantic accessing.

Since he could often begin the written form of a word, PT was encouraged to write as a self-cue. His reading was not strong, suggesting that he was reading via his impaired semantic system. Therefore grapheme–phoneme (letter–sound) conversion skills were also worked on at home with his wife. By 1 year post-onset he was able to read aloud regular CVC words without literal paraphasias, but found the process very distressing. Early exploratory work on sentence structure (using who/doing/what/when/where/how) was abandoned. PT appeared to have difficulty understanding the task.

Retesting at about 18 months post-CVA showed dramatic improvements (Table 3.3.1). He appeared to have established good single word skills, at least for concrete nouns.

Table 3.3.1 Retesting at 18 months post-CVA (all tests drawn from the PALPA)

Spoken word to picture matching test	40/40
Written word to picture matching test	39/40
Spoken naming	32/40 (literal paraphasic errors)
Written naming	39/40

Investigations leading to mapping therapy

Informal observations

By this time PT had had 18 months of single word semantic therapy, and he was very keen to read and write sentences. Although there were still severe word finding difficulties in his spontaneous speech and writing, there were fewer empty fillers and more appropriate content words.

However, well-formed sentences were uncommon. When these did occur, the production seemed uncontrolled and they were rarely repeated.

A closer look at his written sentences revealed interesting strengths and weaknesses (see Table 3.3.2 for examples). PT did seem to be accessing some elements of sentence structure. He was producing many more nouns and some grammatical words, such as determiners, auxiliaries and the occasional verb tense. He also seemed able to produce sentences whose structure did not require multiple mapping. For example he had some success combining one argument with a verb ('Spurs are won today') and could produce the stative construction 'to be' + complement (e.g. 'the coffee was nice'). Table 3.3.2 even shows the successful building of a passive ('the water is put into the kettle').

Table 3.3.2 Examples of written sentences (January 1995)

Spontaneous output

1. Their own to read hat come.
2. Spurs are winning the bad to rifle today.
3. Spurs are won today to reach out the Newcastle.
4. Arsenal with for to reach out till sill to is silly.
5. The Bank although fill that more money is stupid.

Written description of making a cup of coffee

1. The water is put into the kettle, this is learn to boil.
2. The mug is put into the coffee and sugar.
3. The milk was left into the jug.
4. The kettle was boil and the mug was put into the water.
5. The coffee was nice, thank you.

Despite these skills, there were problems with predicate argument structure. For example, reversal errors were seen, in which the nouns were misordered round a verb (e.g. 'the mug is put into the coffee and sugar'). There were also problems with verb retrieval. This resulted in inappropriate verbs being used (e.g. 'Spurs are won today to *reach out* the Newcastle'), and verb omissions. PT's knowledge of the type of arguments required by verbs was variable. He seemed to know that *put* required a goal argument ('The water is put into the kettle'), but also used this type of argument inappropriately with *left* ('The milk was left into the jug').

PT's production seemed influenced by the nature of the event which he was trying to describe. In the 'cup of coffee' examples, PT appeared to have clearly defined and relatively simple events in mind and these sentences contain his most structured output. In the football examples, he attempted some quite complex ideas. For example, in sentence 5, he might be trying to convey that Spurs were planning to change an area of seating, known as 'the Bank', from public to private use in order to raise money. The complexity of this idea plunges his output into jargon. In sentence 2, 'rifle' may be a semantic error for Arsenal, who are known as 'The Gunners'.

From these observations, I hypothesised that PT had access to some elements of sentence structure and mapping, but that this was weak and not under control. PT thought these sentences correct when he gave them to me. In retrospect, it would have been interesting to see his response to them later e.g. in a grammatical judgement task.

Assessments

Tests of sentence comprehension

Several commentators argue that mapping is a central process (e.g. Jones 1986). Therefore a mapping deficit in output should also manifest in input, and in both spoken and written modalities.

In order to probe for this, I tested PT's auditory and written sentence comprehension, using the PALPA Sentence Picture Matching Test (Kay *et al.* 1992). In this test the person hears, or reads a sentence which has to be matched to one of three pictures. The distractor pictures are either reversals, or illustrate incorrect lexical items. A range of sentence forms are tested, including simple actives, passives, comparative adjectives and gapped forms (such as 'The man is demonstrating what to do'). The same stimuli are used in written and auditory tests, though in a different order.

PT's score in the written and spoken modalities was identical (40/60). He also produced a very similar error pattern. He made relatively few errors in simple active sentences or non-reversible sentences where pragmatics helped. He could also immediately dismiss the lexical distractors based on another verb. However, whenever comprehension relied upon mapping knowledge, PT had great difficulties. Thus he was poor with reversible active and passive sentences. He also made several errors in processing **converse relation verbs**, such as 'buy' and 'sell', which are semantically and thematically complex.

PT's comprehension was assessed further with the Jones Test (1984). This is an auditory sentence–picture matching task, with choice from three pictures – the target, a distractor with reverse mapping, and a picture depicting a different lexical verb. The stimuli are all reversible with no pragmatic bias to aid comprehension, e.g. 'The hairdresser shoots the vicar', 'the soldier throws the drummer'. The test includes varying verb types, in order to determine whether comprehension is affected by the semantic complexity of the verb. PT scored 38/60. All his errors involved the selection of the reversal distractor. He was unaffected by the nature of the verb.

Assessment of verb production

PT's ability to produce single verbs was tested. He was presented with 20 Winslow Press Verb Cards: 10 illustrating intransitive or optionally transitive verbs, such as a baby crawling and a man drinking (a cup of tea); and 10 illustrating transitive verbs, such as a woman smelling flowers. They were all familiar action verbs.

The pictures were presented individually and he was asked 'What is he/she doing?' If PT was unable to respond, a sentence closure was used to cue 'He/she is ...?' If this failed he was given a semantic cue, then a phonemic cue, then written information about the first letter or syllable. Unlike post-therapy testing, PT was not asked to produce the full sentence.

The results are shown in Table 3.3.3. This test showed that PT still had weakness in single word verb retrieval, particularly with transitive verbs. The extra thematic information associated with these items may have made retrieval more difficult, even though this information was not required in the task.

Table 3.3.3 Pre-treatment results with Winslow Press Verb Cards

Intransitive/optionally transitive verbs	
5/10	no cueing necessary
2/10	produced after a self-cue in which he wrote the initial letter
3/10	cued by SLT (1 semantic, 2 written syllable)
Transitive verbs	
1/10	no cueing necessary
7/10	cued by SLT (3 semantic and 4 phonemic)
2/10	not accessed

PT appeared to focus on the objects in the pictures, rather than the main event. For example, he might try to describe what the person was looking at rather than what he was doing. Perseverations across items also occurred.

Word class differentiation

Since PT had occasionally produced nouns instead of verbs, I decided to check noun/verb differentiation. He was given 10 simple SV sentences and asked to underline the 'doing' word or verb. He scored 100% very quickly. It seemed that he could distinguish nouns and verbs, although this could have been tested further with more complex sentences.

Assessment summary

PT's production showed some typical signs of a **mapping impairment**. Verb retrieval was impaired, causing omissions and errors. This seemed affected by the number of arguments commanded by a verb, even if he did not have to realise those arguments. Word order was also impaired, with reversal errors and instances of totally anomalous output. The formal comprehension assessments supported the hypothesis that PT had weak mapping skills, since reversal errors were common.

The mapping therapy

Aims

1. By drawing his attention to the syntactic structure of the sentence and the thematic mapping involved, I hoped to provide PT with a cognitive strategy for control over his language processing. He could then use this when on-line spontaneous processing broke down, for both comprehension and expression.
2. Given his own aims, I hoped the therapy would result in improved reading comprehension at sentence level, perhaps allowing PT to read for pleasure.
3. If the hypothesis was correct, and if the therapy materials were accurate in targeting this, I expected PT's performance on the Jones test and PALPA sentence comprehension tests to improve.
4. I also hoped for some signs of improved predicate–argument sentence construction in writing – being slower and more clearly thought out – if not in speech.

A control task was not used for comparison. Identifying an external control task would have been difficult since therapy involved most of the lexical processing systems (input and output, and in both modalities). A non-lexical task, such as non-word reading, was not viable as PT was continuing his grapheme–phoneme conversion exercises.

Therapy regime

Given PT's desire to read, it seemed appropriate to use the written modality for input. Also, PT was keen to take work home. Any gains made in the written modality should generalise to the spoken modality, given the centrality of the mapping process.

Therapy materials were loosely based on Jones's input work with BB (Jones 1986) and consisted of a set of graded sentences for labelling, though PT also initiated some output tasks. The basic progression included identifying the action in SV sentences, identifying the action and agent in SV sentences, identifying the action, agent and theme in SVO sentences. The variables were:

- animacy of agent/theme
- inclusion of non-argument phrases such as prepositional phrases and adverbs
- use of passive
- movement from sentences which could be interpreted 'pragmatically' to those which required word order interpretation.

Verb core semantic complexity was not systematically manipulated.

To prevent 'training' individual verbs rather than the underlying idea, those verbs used in the Jones test and the Winslow Press Verb Cards were avoided in therapy materials.

Cueing took the form of PT drawing the appropriate picture. I considered that this strengthened his semantic accessing, externalised elements of the problem solving and thus allowed more concentration to be channelled into linguistic processing. If this failed, we discussed the sentence, acting it out where appropriate, or simplified the variables, e.g. by providing a pragmatic bias, and working back up to the original sentence in stages.

Originally PT was to read the sentence silently. However, he insisted on reading the sentences aloud as well for auditory confirmation, despite frequent stumblings while retrieving the phonological form.

I also intended that he should underline the correct word in response to questions '**who?**', '**doing?**', '**what?**', but it quickly became obvious he did not understand **wh-** questions. Rather than spend time devising and training symbols, we discussed the terms agent/action/theme at the appropriate stages. These terms were then used to label the sentences, which worked well.

The programme

1. Identify the action in SV sentences: human agent, mixed intransitive/optionally transitive verbs. For example:

   John Major sighed.
   The Queen sneezed.

PT managed this very quickly with 100% accuracy. I had tried to introduce the idea of '**who**', but this was quickly abandoned.

2. Identify the action and agent in SV sentences: animate agent, mixed intransitive/optionally transitive verbs. For example:

   My grandfather snores.
   The parrot swore.

PT found these a little more difficult. I encouraged him to read the sentence word by word (aloud if necessary), repeat the whole sentence, think about the picture in his head, draw it if necessary, and then say the sentence again, hopefully driven by the picture. I suspected that he was having difficulty with lexical semantics, rather than in differentiating the agent and action.

3. Identify the agent and action in SV sentences: more complex noun phrases. For example:

   The little grey mouse escaped.
   The little old lady in the corner chuckled.

Surprisingly, PT quickly identified the NP/VP constituent boundary, though he expressed concern that there appeared to be groups within the 'agent', and wanted to know why!

4. Production of SV sentences to describe pictures of a single action. For example:

   The girl is laughing.
   The boy is jumping.

PT accessed the verb, then wrote it; accessed the noun for the agent and wrote it; constructed the sentence, then read the sentence aloud and checked it with the picture. This was a big jump into an output task. However, PT initiated this, saying he wanted to produce some sentences himself. PT included the definite article *the* in the noun phrase and verb morphemes without prompting.

5. Identify the agent and action in SV sentences: animate agents, complex NPs, additional non-arguments (e.g. adverbs, past participles). For example:

   The greedy schoolboy burped loudly.
   The fat burglar tiptoed past.

PT made a clear distinction between NP and VP, but was less happy with the random non-argument structures, wanting a label for these too. We discussed them generally as 'extra information'.

6. Introduction of theme – the concept was discussed, followed by identification of agent, action and theme in SVO sentences: simple NPs, simple VP, animate agent, inanimate theme, pragmatically biased. For example:

   The bride cut the cake.
   The cat drank the milk.

There were no problems here.

7. PT to change the above sentences into the passive: animate agent, inanimate theme, pragmatically biased. For example:

> The cake was cut by the bride.
> The milk was drunk by the cat.

Again this was another big jump, but I wanted to ensure PT was understanding the thematic roles rather than using syntactic position. PT drew the picture which went with the active sentence (*The bride cut the cake*). Then we focused on *cake*, and began the written sentence with it, wrote the verb *cut*, then *the bride*. I then asked PT to draw the picture which corresponded with this sentence, which he did with great difficulty. This led to a discussion that other words (*be* and *by*) were necessary to prevent the first picture changing to the second (*cake cut bride*), and we added these in the appropriate positions, together with identifying thematic labels (*The cake was cut by the bride*). PT quickly picked up the syntactic and thematic patterning.

8. Production of SVO sentences using family photographs as stimuli, method as in 4. For example:

> L is watering the flowers.
> The girls are watching Caspar [the cat] in the garden.

Again, PT initiated this activity. Family photographs made the task more personally relevant, and hopefully more likely to carry over. The trade-off was that stimuli were less easy to control for variables; PT also had to interpret the event and choose a perspective. Since there was often more than one event happening in the picture, PT found it difficult to focus upon one alone, or to interpret a combination of actions as one main event (e.g. the girls are watching Caspar, the girls are standing on the path, the girls are in the garden, Caspar is playing with the string, etc). To overcome this, PT was encouraged to retrieve all the relevant lexical items, including verbs. He was then asked to choose a verb, point to the activity, then pick out the arguments from the lexical items already retrieved. He then ordered these into a sentence, making the necessary morphological changes if he could.

Having retrieved the lexical items, PT did seem able to choose appropriate arguments given the semantic requirements of the verb, which surprised me. He then very quickly mapped these syntactically. PT found this one of the most enjoyable therapy tasks.

9. Identification of agent, action and theme in SVO sentences: animate agents and themes, pragmatically biased. For example:

The barber shaved the customer.
The vicar preached a very long sermon.

PT drew the picture corresponding with the active sentence, then changed the sentence into the passive as in 7, checking that the picture had not changed. This took time, but there were no consistent problems.

10. Production of mixed SV and SVO sentences to pictures (not passives), as in 4. For example:

The man is sleeping.
The man is combing his hair.

PT wanted to know why some actions had themes and some did not. This suggested that although PT had grasped a pattern with the written stimuli, he had not fully understood the need for arguments or their role around the individual verbs.

By providing the written stimuli for labelling I had presented the appropriate number of arguments each time without checking PT had access to or appreciated this information. We could have checked sentence acceptability at this stage. Instead, I attempted to answer his question by discussing intransitive, optionally transitive and transitive verb structures!

We also very briefly looked at how the thematic role changes in some optionally transitive verbs (e.g. *the door opened, the man opened the door*). Although it seems rather complex, PT was asking the questions, and he appeared to understand and enjoy the patterning.

At this time PT attempted spontaneous written sentences at home, similar to those used in therapy (e.g. *the cat chased the dog/the dog was chased by the cat*). This suggested he was remembering structures but not generating them himself. PT then became muddled (e.g. *the hospital is big/big is by the hospital*). He knew the sentence was incorrect, and wanted to know why the agent/action/theme structure did not work.

Despite correct responses in therapy tasks, it seemed that PT did not have a clear grasp of agent and theme. We discussed the roles again, acting out the thematic roles (loosely interpreted) e.g. *PT thumped Susan, Susan thumped PT*.

We also discussed how these **action sentences** are only one type of sentence construction, and that he already seemed able to produce successful **description sentences** (e.g. *the coffee is nice*).

11. Recap identifying agent, action and theme in active then passive sentences: animate agents, inanimate themes, pragmatic bias. For example:

The bees make honey.
Honey is made by the bees.

PT drew the picture, then labelled it. He then labelled the constituents in the sentence, whether active or passive in relation to the picture. PT appeared to find this too easy. When left alone he skipped drawing the pictures and immediately labelled the sentences.

12. PT to insert an appropriate agent into a given SVO sentence frame: animate agents, pragmatic bias, no picture stimulus. For example:

> *The barber* cuts hair.
> *The policeman* directs the traffic.

PT found this very difficult. He seemed to have difficulty with verb core semantics and interpretation of the event. At first he tried to ignore the verb and produced a noun associated with the second argument, but not necessarily appropriate as an agent for the given verb. When this happened, I drew PT's attention to the verb again, and encouraged him to draw a picture of the event, which he usually managed to do successfully, including an appropriate agent. We then discussed who the agent PT had drawn was likely to be, and completed the task. Again, PT's initial response of an associated rather than an appropriate noun suggested the concept of 'agent' was still fragile.

13. PT to insert an appropriate agent into a given intransitive SV + PP sentence frame: animate agent, pragmatic bias. For example:

> *The old man* is sitting in the armchair.
> *The soldiers* are marching down the road.

Given the problems in the previous task, this was rather ambitious. The non-argument preposition phrases were included to give contextual information for a likely verb. On reflection, although transitive verbs were usually more difficult for PT to retrieve, the information provided by the theme argument would probably have given more immediate context. PT was unable to identify a linking action from the written stimuli alone. I encouraged him to draw separate pictures of the agent and the preposition phrase noun, then to draw another picture with them integrated into a likely event. He found this easier. Once he had drawn this event, he had no problems identifying the action – he could act it out – and the task became one of lexical retrieval.

14. Identify the agent, action and theme in given sentences: the stimuli progressed from 'pragmatically interpretable' to reversible sentences, using the same verb. Both actives and passives were included. For example:

> The footballer kicked the ball.
> The naughty boy kicked the dog.

The very naughty boy kicked his granny.
The ball was kicked by the footballer.
The poor dog was kicked by the naughty boy.
The very poor granny was kicked by the very naughty boy.

(See Figure 3.3.1). PT drew the picture for the sentence, labelled the thematic roles in the picture then labelled the sentence. There were no difficulties.

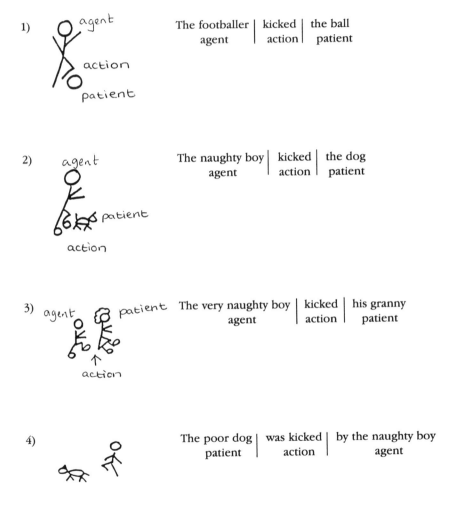

1) The footballer | kicked | the ball
    agent | action | patient

2) The naughty boy | kicked | the dog
    agent | action | patient

3) The very naughty boy | kicked | his granny
    agent | action | patient

4) The poor dog | was kicked | by the naughty boy
    patient | action | agent

Figure 3.3.1 Example of mapping therapy materials: Task 14.

15. PT to produce SVO sentence to describe line drawings of single events: human agents, inanimate themes. For example:

The boy is climbing a tree.
The man is driving a car.

Prompts (originally **who?**, **doing?**, **what?**) were relabelled **agent?**, **action?**, **theme?**. PT had to identify the arguments in the picture and retrieve the lexical forms. He then used these to construct the sentence. PT managed this quickly, apart from verb retrieval difficulties.

16. PT to produce SVO sentence to given picture stimuli: the pictures consisted of drawings of two objects, representing argument nouns, separated by a written cue 'VERB'. An instrument was also drawn to cue the verb. For example:

(drawing of a woman)   (drawing of a knife)   (drawing of bread)
VERB

PT was required to label the three noun phrases, use the instrument to retrieve an appropriate verb and construct the sentence. Again, even after retrieving the names of the given items, PT found it hard to conceptualise a likely event. He was encouraged to draw a picture combining all three arguments, which he usually managed successfully. Once he had done this, he had little difficulty identifying the action concept, though there were still difficulties with retrieval of the lexical form of the verb. Having found the verb, he quickly constructed an appropriate sentence, but made occasional errors mixing the theme with the instrument. Providing the syntactic frame: 'with the ...' reduced these errors.

17. As 16 but with two argument NPs and an instrument in random order on page. For example:

(picture of a knife)   (picture of a cake)   (picture of a woman)

PT noticed that the order was random, but then tried to construct sentences using the given order. I was not sure whether this suggested weak semantics, or a general compliance on his part with the vagaries of speech therapy material. Once again he had difficulty distinguishing the likely instrument from the theme and as before he was helped by drawing the overall event. This enabled him to label the arguments, search for the verb and construct the sentence. He incorporated the instrument using the **with** prepositional phrase. A future marker was spontaneously produced for some items (*The woman will cut the cake with the knife*).

18. PT to produce SV(O) sentences in response to photographic sequences. For example:

The girl kicks the boy.
The boy is crying.
The mum is telling off the girl.

Again, with the realistic detail, PT found it hard to focus on one action within the picture. To break the task down, PT named items within each picture, including verbs, as brainstorming exercise. He then acted out the picture to pick out the main event, which he did successfully on most occasions. Having focused on this event, PT found the sentence construction from the previously accessed words relatively easy. He rapidly progressed to extended sequences of up to six pictures.

Therapy outcomes

PT's responses to the therapy materials had been promising. The verb accessing had been hard, but identification of the thematic roles and his ordering of thematic roles in production appeared consistent. After 10 months of mapping therapy the pre-therapy assessments were re-administered.

Tests of sentence comprehension

The Jones Picture Selection Test (spoken and written) and the written PALPA Sentence Picture Matching Test were re-administered. In all cases, PT was unable to perform the task, and the tests were abandoned after a few items (The PALPA Spoken Sentence Picture Matching Test was not attempted).

Assessment of verb production

PT's verb retrieval was tested using the Winslow Press Verb Cards. Now PT was also asked to compose a sentence in response to the stimuli. The cueing hierarchy was as previously but without sentence closure. See Table 3.3.4.

Discussion of post-therapy tests

Looking at the verb retrieval test first, the number spontaneously accessed was disappointing in both the intransitive and transitive groups. However, PT self-cued more effectively and the number of verbs achieved independently, with or without self-cueing, rose from 8 to 13.

Table 3.3.4 Post-treatment results with Winslow Press Verb Cards

	Baseline (Jan 1995)	Re-test (Dec 1995)
Intrans/opt transitive verbs		
no cueing necessary	5/10	4/10
self-cue	2/10	4/10
cued by SLT	3/10	2/10
Transitive verbs		
no cueing necessary	1/10	0/10
self-cued	0/10	5/10
cued by SLT	7/10	5/10
not accessed	2/10	

The main surprise was PT's method of self-cueing. Even before I had mentioned production of the full sentence, he used sentence construction as a strategy. With the intransitive verbs he produced the subject noun phrase with appropriate intonation several times to retrieve the verb (previous self-cueing had been finger writing). With the transitive verbs, spontaneous self-cueing included: acting the event; using the second argument as a stepping stone to the verb (e.g. 'Not the radio – listening'); and using an intoned sentence frame with a gap for the verb ('The man is ... the orange').

As soon as PT had retrieved the verb he quickly produced the full sentence spontaneously (spoken output). He made only two sentence errors, both of which involved mapping the wrong argument after the verb (e.g. 'The woman is cutting the scissors') and both of which were quickly self-corrected.

PT's performance on the sentence comprehension tests was very disappointing. This was clearly not due to the modality of presentation, given the equally disastrous performance on the Jones test in both the written and spoken format. PT may have been influenced by the nature of the verbs used in the tests, which were lower in frequency and more semantically complex than those used during therapy. For example, unlike the tests, the therapy stimuli did not include directional motion verbs (such as 'follow'), or converse relation verbs (such as 'buy').

I asked PT for his thoughts. In the Jones Picture Selection Test, he reported that the detail in the line drawings appeared to be triggering other words in his head, causing difficulty focusing on the main action and requiring much monitoring and inhibiting. For example, assessment took place in a session after we had used NP instruments in therapy materials to suggest an action. The people in the pictures all hold 'instruments' to identify their professions, many of which are unrelated to the event. PT knew that these instruments were not connected with the event in question, but found their presence confusing, and heard himself retrieving the associated verb.

When asked about the PALPA sentence comprehension, PT replied that many of the sentences did not seem to have agent/action/theme, so he did not know what to do. He was no longer happy to guess, as he had done prior to therapy.

Informal comprehension task

The insight that PT was no longer prepared to risk failure in a formal comprehension test suggested that a less formal, more naturalistic comprehension task was needed to probe for any acquired mapping skills. Accordingly, I gave PT written statements to interpret and comment on (April 1996). All statements involved complex reversible semantic relations (see Table 3.3.5). These examples show that, although hesitant, PT could access the semantics of the verbs and was aware of the roles played by the arguments within the event. This information must have been derived from the linguistic structure, given the reversibility of the sentences and the inclusion of a false statement. It seemed as if some comprehension gains had taken place, which were obscured by other difficulties with the formal tests.

Table 3.3.5 Examples used in the informal comprehension test

Tony Blair will beat John Major at the next election
S: Do you think that this is true?
P: So he (pointing to TB) is going to win?
S: Yep ... do you think that's true?
P: At the moment, yeah ...

The Allies defeated the Germans at Dunkirk
S: Is that true?
P: Um – if there was nothing there (covering up 'at Dunkirk') – she – that was in 1945, they won (pointing to the Allies), but there? (pointing to 'Dunkirk')
P: ...you see, if the – the Allies was Dunkirk, so everyone's – they're ok – no, they lost there!
P: 'The Allies ... defeated the Germans at Dunkirk', then that would've been after, when, you know, its either 1944 or 1945.

PT's output during the task also shows some progress. We might, for example, compare his production here to his pre-therapy problems with the verb *beat* in the football sentences see Table 3.3.2.

Generalisation to spontaneous speech

Although I had hoped therapy would provide PT with a cognitive strategy for controlling his output, there is no evidence that he spontaneously used the strategy when losing control of sentence structure in speech.

The cognitive load in production, requiring both mapping and lexical retrieval, was perhaps too great for him.

In addition, much of what PT wished to say was not easily translated into a simple agent/action/theme structure. Advice often given – to simplify a message to fit available structure – perhaps did not acknowledge the complexity of the task.

Generalisations to reading

After therapy, PT began to read books, almost for pleasure. After much searching, we found a series of picture based books with an appropriate story line, and just two or three sentences per picture.

Although PT could access semantics through silent reading, he preferred to read aloud for the additional auditory input. On first reading, PT's intonation suggested that he was working at the level of individual lexical semantics. Once the sentence was completed, he usually re-read it to ensure comprehension. He was then able to relate the events to the picture, pointing out the relevant phrases and using the events described to work out the identity of new characters.

Generalisations to writing

PT produced this written description after about 7 months of mapping therapy (October 1995). It was produced at home, unsolicited and unaided.

> Morning, six o clock it went wrong. 28 August 1993. my Dad his birthday. Stroke I went to sleep. Saturday. Sunday. Monday and Tuesday. I slept 4 days. My eyes went wrong. L, L, K, Mum + Dad K, N and Grandad, P the girl. The G and A, I + C*. The cried away one waiting. Every one I cried and cried. A Wednesday the blood went out. The lou were wrong and I want to see the nurse, so I can't to me with the rights. The right leg and arm didn't work. The left leg and arm were ok. The lou were funny and didn't start so I pulled out so I left it out. The blood were every were.

(NB. * Names given in full in the original; 'lou' = catheter)

Although clear problems remain, this passage shows some skills. At paragraph level there is sequential structure. At sentence level, despite morpheme difficulties, difficulties with grammatical words and difficulties with verb retrieval, the passage is semantically coherent. The passage communicates the intended message quite successfully.

Given our therapy, there were surprisingly few agent/action/theme constructions, but most of the verbs PT had accessed (*go, sleep, cry, want, can, work, start*) do not require an agent and a theme. In the penultimate sentence PT omits the theme with *pull* but includes the theme with *leave*. Most of the sentences have a definite syntactic shape, with evidence of quite complex verb structure, e.g. want + infinitive.

PT made further attempts to apply the skills learnt in therapy in his writing. He was encouraged to focus primarily on highly imageable action events, which could be described using the agent / action / theme structure. This led to a number of successful written descriptions of the actions of family members. These attempts were executed independently at home (May/June 1996):

L is cutting the chicken for the pasta
L is washing the mushrooms
L is chopping the onions and the bacon
L is drinking the wine
L is putting the mushroom, bacon and onion onto the fry pan
L is boiling the water
L is weighing the pasta
The water is boiling, the pasta is putting into the bowl.
Everything is ready to eat.
L is painting the soldiers
K is reading the books
Grandad has to go to the Doctor for the X-Ray
I would like a nice cup of tea, please
L is putting the washing in the machine washing
We walked to the shops, and we the sun
I peeled the potatoe
I painted the fence today.

Conclusions

This experience of mapping therapy with PT raised more questions than definite conclusions.

Did PT initially have a mapping problem?

At outset PT demonstrated classic mapping symptoms in input and output, and in the written and spoken modalities. The formal assessments seemed to support the hypothesis.

In retrospect, many of the symptoms could have been the result of weak verb core semantics rather than difficulties with the associated mapping. Further investigations into his general verb processing pre-therapy would have been helpful. These tasks might have included verb selection against distractors to check verb core semantics, and judgement tasks in which he had to judge the number of arguments demanded by a verb, and the semantic features of those arguments.

Whether the therapy strengthened a weakness, or developed an emerging strength given increasing verb accessing, perhaps remains unclear.

What went wrong in the sentence comprehension assessments?

Hypothesising a weakness in verb core semantics may account for the discrepancy in performance between the therapy materials and the assessments.

PT later revealed that in the pre-therapy comprehension tests he had tried to link the individual words with elements found within the pictures, rather than understand the sentences. He had been guessing, and had little sense of a picture being correct. With increased awareness post-therapy, PT was less willing to commit himself when he knew there was the possibility of working out the answer.

We had practised much lexical retrieval as a precursor to sentence construction, and so accessing seems to have increased. With this, unwanted stimuli appeared to be triggering meanings and lexical forms which PT had to monitor and inhibit. Thus, as PT's language skills increased, more monitoring was required. The written stimuli used in therapy contained fewer distractors than the detailed pictures of the tests.

Have PT's language skills and communication changed in response to the therapy?

Although formal assessment results were disappointing, PT's communicative abilities did appear to change.

His speech still displayed marked word finding difficulties, though possibly not to the same extent. Although PT was not recorded pre-therapy, and so comparison cannot be made, his output post-therapy seemed to have more sentence structure. He still used filler phrases ('you know'), but there were no instances of jargon. He monitored well. As a result his output was relevant and he attempted to correct lexical errors. His selfcueing strategies in the verb retrieval test suggested that PT was deriving extra information from sentence structure to help word retrieval.

Pre-therapy PT's written output was highly error prone; post-therapy he was able to construct simple sentences much more consistently and independently. This was becoming a source of satisfaction to him.

The beginning of sentence comprehension from linguistic analysis, rather than lexical and contextual cues, was a major achievement for PT. The possibility of reading some of his own books again – even if only scanning – was not quite so remote. Also, there was potential to use sentence level material more meaningfully in therapy, even if working on single word level semantics.

Was the therapy mapping therapy – what did it do, and how did it work?

Therapy aimed to make the mapping processes cognitively explicit, and in particular, how the roles of agent and theme are mapped on to active and passive sentences. One important device for achieving this aim was the use of drawings as a first stage in generating output. These drawings demonstrated clearly who was initiating the action and hence helped to differentiate the roles of agent and theme.

It is possible that the therapy tasks and the way they were used also:

• increased single word semantics, especially for verbs
• increased PT's awareness of event structure, at a more abstract level
• increased PT's cognitive awareness of general sentence structure, including mapping, which has enabled him to impose a level of control on his fluent output, and construct more sentence semantics in input; PT now reads aloud with appropriate sentence intonation
• encouraged him to focus on meaning when reading aloud, and with increased semantic drive accessing the phonological form become more consistent.

However, given his sentence comprehension difficulties, his early attempts at structure and his wishes regarding reading and writing, I think mapping was an appropriate target for therapy.

What next?

After the mapping programme, therapy focused on increasing the verb core semantics which had been highlighted in the mapping therapy. Our hypothesis was that increased semantic drive would reduce word finding difficulties in both written and spoken modalities, and enable PT to take advantage of his improved sentence level processing skills.

Tasks included input and output tasks – verb grading, verb choice with close semantic distractors, sentence–picture judgement tasks etc. While keeping the focus of therapy on input, PT was keen to output, so these judgements were incorporated into simple sentence output tasks.

Giving PT the opportunity to express fears within a safe environment was a continuing feature of therapy. At the time of writing, he has much to come to terms with. There is much work to do.

Acknowledgements

I would like to thank Eirian Jones for her infectious enthusiasm and for her comments on the paper. I would also like to thank my colleague Morag Bixley, PT's therapist for the first year, for access to her notes and for her comments on the paper.

I am also indebted to Professor Paul Fletcher for helpful soccer insights into the written sentences in Table 3.3.2.

Chapter 3.4
Afterword

JANE MARSHALL

The patients described in this section shared a number of similarities. Both had severe problems producing sentences despite relative skills in single word comprehension and production. Furthermore, there was quite a lot of evidence that their difficulties were not primarily syntactic. Even before therapy, their output contained a number of syntactic features. For example, although Gordon could not generate verb structures he could realise the syntactic elements of noun phrases, such as determiners and inflections and, while much of PT's output was anomalous, some sophisticated forms, such as passives, were seen. Further evidence emerged during therapy. One component of the treatment required the patients to segment written sentences into their constituent phrases. Both patients had no problems with this task, suggesting that their intuitions about the syntactic structures of sentences were largely intact. Pethers also comments that PT spontaneously supplied verb morphology during therapy production tasks.

Such similarities encouraged the authors to reach similar processing 'diagnoses'. They both concluded that their patients had a semantic level deficit. In particular, they identified problems in verb retrieval and in building semantic representations which specify the relationship between the verb and its arguments. These 'diagnoses', in turn, motivated strikingly similar therapy programmes, both of which borrowed heavily from the mapping treatment developed by Jones (1986).

Yet how similar were Gordon and PT? One obvious point of contrast was their comprehension, in that Gordon never showed any difficulties understanding sentences, including semantically reversible ones, whereas PT did. They also responded very differently to the therapy. Gordon made rapid and extensive progress, particularly in his production of verbs and verb structures. Furthermore, some of his gains went beyond the aims of the treatment. For example, additional syntactic features emerged, such as pronouns and verb inflections, despite not being specifically targeted. PT's gains were more difficult to detect, although progress seemed to occur in production and some informal comprehension tasks. PT also encountered a number of difficulties during the treatment, particularly when he was asked to produce a verb. Interestingly, additional non-verbal processing of events, i.e. through the medium of drawing, was helpful here.

Interpreting different responses to therapy is very difficult, not least because there were substantial differences between the programmes. However, taken with the comprehension evidence, the outcomes might suggest that PT's and Gordon's problems were, in fact, quite different. We might speculate, rather as Bryan does, that Gordon had considerable semantic knowledge about verbs at the outset. For some reason, he was apparently unable to recruit this knowledge for production, possibly because delayed semantic processing interacted with residual problems in phonological retrieval. PT's difficulties were perhaps more profound. As Pethers comments, he may need much more help in processing the semantic features of verbs and events, before major improvements in production can be achieved.

We should not be surprised by these differences. Other studies have found that subjects with apparently similar deficits responded very differently to the same treatments, and that these varying responses, in part, reflected important variations in the language resources available to the individuals (Byng *et al*. 1994). It seems that our mechanisms for 'diagnosing' language deficits are still very crude. Even if we can pin down the likely level of impairment, subtle fractionations within that level may still be obscured. Researchers delight in such subtleties, but hard-pressed clinicians probably find them something of a pain in the neck. They have to respond to their patient's difficulties here and now, even if our understanding of those difficulties is only partial. Yet all is not lost. Providing therapy is pitched at the right general level of processing, some of the finer individual variations can emerge on the hoof. Indeed, we saw that, with PT, language testing became *less* informative with time, as he became more reluctant to risk failure. Therefore, for him, possibly the only medium which could illuminate his problems further was therapy.

Part 4
Pragmatics: a breakdown in contextual meaning

Chapter 4.1
Introduction

JAMES LAW

...The purpose of the elephant has got to be respected ...

Is it possible to speak of pragmatic disability in the same breath as deficits affecting phonological, lexical and syntactic processing? The answer, of course, depends on how we construe pragmatics. There has been a tendency to describe it as meaning which goes beyond the structural properties of an utterance. This 'wastebasket' analogy (McTear and Conti-Ramsden 1992) may make some sort of sense as far as we are able to exclude contextual information from our understanding of structure, but it is not very helpful in explaining what we mean by a pragmatic disorder. It may be more useful to pick out a number of levels on which it is possible to examine contextual meaning. As with the discussion of processing in earlier sections in this book it is possible to draw a distinction between **input** and **output** at each level.

The first is the **suprasegmental level**. The listener has to perceive not only the combination of phonemes which go to make up words but must also detect the way intonation and stress is used to modify meaning. Commonly used examples include interrogative and imperative forms but intention is also conveyed through more subtle modifications such as those associated with irony and sarcasm, changes which children and adults with language disorders often find difficult to decode. There is clearly a developmental dimension here because children who are not experiencing problems acquiring language often struggle with this type of meaning well into the school years and indeed some adults are naturally more adept at interpreting meaning at this level. Nevertheless by the time children reach the age of 6, most have developed a keen understanding of a speaker's intentions as determined by the **way** in which something is said rather than by **what** is said. On the output side, even young children formulate and convey intention through prosodic structure but this is probably more apparent in adults who rely heavily on the non-linguistic aspect of the interaction to convey meaning. In the final analysis it may be less a matter of whether one group relies more or less heavily on intonation but whether children and adults rely on it for different purposes.

A second level refers to the way in which the context impinges on the structural aspects of linguistic form. Although it may be possible to decode an utterance from its lexical and syntactic properties alone, more commonly it is necessary to go beyond the immediate structure to interpret fully its meaning. For example to interpret diectic or anaphoric relationships it is necessary for the listener to refer to factors beyond the structure of the utterance. Take the following utterance:

> He boasted that the one that he had caught had been this big.

This is adequate as a sentence but is impossible to understand fully without a wealth of supplementary information. Likewise, to encode such meanings may be fairly straightforward but to encode them such that the listener is able to detect the intended emphasis often leads to difficulties. This is especially true between communicative partners who for social or personal reasons do not share the same communicative assumptions. Another layer here is the use of metaphor. Invariably this involves the listener making associations in order to extract the appropriate meaning. In some cases the metaphor may be very common, sometimes taking the from of 'frozen' or 'dead' metaphors such as 'life is a bowl of cherries' or 'it's raining cats and dogs'. More familiar metaphors may be easier to decode but this type of utterance often proves problematic for listeners struggling with pragmatic skills.

A third level refers to the need for speaker and listener to establish shared meaning for communication to take place effectively. If a speaker says

> It's freezing.

there are various ways that such a sentence could be decoded, again according to the context. The appropriate response could be 'yes, it is isn't it' or 'I'll just close the window' or 'no, its your turn to go to the shops!'. The speech act has to be translated between speaker and listener. The **locutionary force** (the meaning conveyed by the structure of the utterance) may be distinct from both the **illocutionary force** (the intended meaning) and the **perlocutionary force** (the perceived meaning) of an utterance. If the intention and the effect do not correspond, speaker and listener are likely to draw inferences or implications about each other's intentions (Grice 1975). For example, if the speaker talks incessantly and does not give the listener an opportunity to enter the conversation it has been suggested that the listener determines that the speaker has broken what Grice terms the 'maxim of quantity' and this leads to judgements about the reason for this. Likewise, if the speaker does not stick to the point and provides unnecessary or patently erroneous information the listener has to judge how to respond and this judgement involves information not related to the structure of language as such. At the heart of this issue is the concept of **relevance** (Sperber and Wilson 1986). For an utterance to work it must have a comparable relevance to both partners and both speaker and listener have to be prepared to negotiate this relevance during the course of the interaction.

A fourth level occurs in the structure of the conversation itself. So for example the conversation may break down because of a misunderstanding of intended meaning. This in itself is a common enough occurrence. Those involved must then renegotiate or repair meanings if the conversation is to continue. This requires careful online monitoring of the other participant's role. Likewise there is a series of rules governing the sequence of conversation which must be mastered if the conversation is to function effectively. For example the individual must learn how to get into conversations, and how to extricate him/herself from them and must be aware, albeit unconsciously, of how these formulaic sequences or what are sometimes known as **adjacency pairs** work.

Although it is possible to see interaction as being a product of linguistic or discourse skills, it also possible that it is more a reflection of the individual's capacity to relate effectively to others. It may be this, more central, capacity which underpins pragmatic skills. This takes us to our fifth and final level. Exactly what this capacity is has been the topic of debate. Some would see it as an affective function, others as a function of social cognition. The latter has received particular attention recently because of the development of theories related to 'theory of mind'. Although considerable progress has been made in this area, and it is clear that those with difficulties in understanding that others have minds will certainly struggle in interpreting intentionality, it is less clear how theory of mind operates in the normal population. Not everyone is equally good at interpreting a speaker's intention, but few have a formally identifiable problem with what have become known as **theory of mind** tasks. Likewise it is not altogether clear how an individual's ability to understand theory of mind can be separated from the ability to understand emotional states in others (Hobson 1993).

To what extent are these levels of pragmatic processing discrete and to what extent do they interact? It seems reasonable to suggest that they interact but in different ways. It is probable that poor understanding of another's intentions will affect the capacity to decode all levels of intended meaning. But it would also be true to say that an individual might have a more discrete problem with interpreting intonation and make errors interpreting the gist of a conversation without it being true that he or she was not able to understand intention completely. Equally it is reasonable to assume that an individual might be inefficient in negotiating the complexities of conversational structure without necessarily having difficulties processing prosodic information or attributing to others thought processes different from his/her own.

It might be argued that problems with pragmatics are really the inevitable consequence of poor language processing and attentional difficulties, that if you have difficulties with online linguistic processing you are likely to have difficulties with the more intricate elements of conversation. This has been shown to be the case both for children with developmental language impairments (Gallagher 1991) and for adults with acquired language impairments (Lesser and Milroy 1993, Lesser and Algar 1995). But this is not necessarily the case. Bishop and Adams (1989), for example, have shown that the capacity of children with specific language impairment to perform referential communication tasks was not necessarily related to their conversational ability. Sacks provides a lovely example of the relative strengths exhibited by some dysphasic patients in this area. In his book *The Man who Mistook his Wife for a Hat* (Sacks 1985) he describes a room full of aphasic patients roaring with laughter over the president's speech, precisely because their pragmatic skills enabled them to see right through the meaning he is conveying in sentence structures that he is using. Sacks comments:

> One cannot lie to an aphasic. He cannot grasp your words, and so cannot be deceived by them, but what he grasps he grasps with infallible precision, namely the expression that goes with the words.

Although Sacks is probably overstating the case, it is possible that both children and adults can have intact pragmatic skills relative to marked problems with the more formal aspects of language processing.

If it is possible for language impaired clients to be more or less impaired pragmatically, is it also possible for people to have pragmatic disorders in isolation? In developmental terms the most commonly reported examples of this phenomenon are autistic children for whom syntactic and phonological form may be retained and who are often able to make judgements about syntactic appropropriateness but who experience difficulties at all the levels outlined above. The same is true to some extent of children with less pronounced problems who are more likely to be labelled as having language impairments. The most common examples are children with Asperger's syndrome or semantic pragmatic disorder. Again their performance is marked by poor interaction skills and relatively intact linguistic skills. In addition many exhibit poor eye contact which will inevitably adversely affect the interaction. It is worth adding a caveat that, although there may be an imbalance in favour of relatively intact grammatical structure in these cases, many use language in quite a formulaic way, peppering their output with learned expressions such as 'by the way ...' or 'well, anyway ...' Although a pragmatic deficit may be associated with other difficulties in communication, it is clear that the disability is sufficiently discrete to merit some level of independent status.

In the case of acquired language disorders there is evidence that individuals with right hemisphere lesions are more vulnerable to pragmatic disability than patients with left hemisphere damage. They have been shown to have comparable structural problems but significantly worse pragmatic skills as marked by the interpetation of metaphor and inferred meaning and by their capacity to retain coherence in discourse (Bryan 1988). Of particular interest here is the fact that such clients commonly are unable to recognise the nature of their difficulties. The brain damage appears to lead to an inability to self-monitor and reflect on the process of communication.

It is reasonable to suggest three possible routes for the potential breakdown in processing. It is plausible that difficulties in decoding context lead to linguistic difficulties, or that linguistic difficulties lead to difficulties in the interaction or that difficulties in the two domains simply co-vary as they do in the normal population. The first of these seems to be particularly likely in the case of children where it is possible to identify a breakdown in shared meaning from a very early stage in the child's development. The child does not focus on the adults around him and does not learn to monitor the external aspects of joint reference – facial expression, prosody, etc. This may be a function of specific processing difficulties or may be affectively determined. Joint referencing becomes a more laborious process as a result and with that comes a poorly developed potential for word and sentence mapping and the ensuing delays may then compound one another. There seems to be some evidence that severely neglected children have problems of this form although their interaction is usually marked by inefficient interaction rather than the type of bizarre output characteristically noted in cases of pragmatic disability. The clearest evidence for this type of route would be finding a dissociation between linguistic and pragmatic skills. Such children would have well developed syntax relative to marked deficits in pragmatics. Although such cases do exist they are probably relatively rare.

If there is no evidence of interaction difficulties in the case history it might be reasonable to assume that the pragmatic deficit was secondary to the other areas of linguistic impairment such as local phonological, syntactic or semantic problems. This would predict that pragmatic disbilities should be present for all language impaired individuals. Although there is a tendency for this to be the case there are many children with syntactic or phonological difficulties who retain intact pragmatic skills. In fact the strongest association here is likely to be between the child's semantic system and their pragmatic abilities. It is difficult to see how these two systems can be completely separate since the establishment of word and sentence meaning depends on sharing the perspective on the world adopted by both speakers.

It might also be that the two domains of language and interactive ability or pragmatics are relatively independent of one another such that problems may or may not co-occur. For example we may encounter a child with very real pragmatic difficulties but no structural linguistic difficulties, or vice versa. Conversely, individuals might have marked disability in both areas. This last possibility seems the most plausible even though we might not expect to find the two functions operating entirely independently of each other. For example, it seems likely that with increased involvement of the child's semantic input system pragmatic functions are likely to be affected.

The interaction between linguistic and pragmatic skills for the adult aphasic client is likely to be rather different. It is easy to see that the language impairment itself is likely to make the individual's capacity to interact with others less efficient. However, it is not clear how far the effects go or how this might change with time. Does the individual become less efficient at interacting as the length of time since the stroke increases? Do the individual's interaction skills deteriorate with time? The answer to these questions seems to be no, suggesting that linguistic impairments do not have a progressive negative impact on pragmatic skills for the adult in the way that they may do for the child. Similarly it is unlikely that pragmatic inpairments in adults will lead to formulation problems as such, although the two may co-occur. The suggestion is, then, that although there may be pragmatic sequelae of left brain damage, the clearest presentations are likely to be a function of right brain lesions, and that linguistic and pragmatic skills will not co-vary in such an unpredictable fashion as they do in the paediatric population.

Having established the need to examine pragmatic skills it is then necessary to identify the best method of accessing them. A number of assessments of the more formal aspects of pragmatics have been developed over the years but their application often proves problematic. Although it is possible to give an individual judgement tasks related to pragmatic abilities it is questionable whether these really reflect what goes on when we make a judgement about the appropriateness of a given utterance, especially when we make those judements in the context of a conversation. In part it is the 'online' nature of pragmatic processing in which the context is continually being monitored which makes formal assessment so difficult. It is possible to test some aspects of appropriateness in behaviour and conversation. Likewise it is possible to judge an individual's capacity to cope with metaphor or some of the more abstract levels of language processing. Language sampling can provide some useful information about the way in which the individual copes with the demands of a conversation. This may be in open ended communication or within the more circumscribed format of recon-structed narratives. **Conversation analysis** has become increasingly popular as a framework for investigating spontaneous communication. Here the linguistic context is reported in full and the role of the inter-locutor explored in the same way as that of the subject. However, even conversational analysis does not capture all of the additional non-verbal information which goes towards informing the pragmatic judgement.

There are a great many ways of approaching intervention for this group of clients because the presenting features may be many and varied. Whatever approach is adopted, it will only work if the individual has developed the capacity to reflect both on their own conversational ability and on the inner states of conversational partners. This **meta-awareness** can be a central issue for adults with right hemisphere lesions and may become the main focus of the intervention. We may not expect such awareness of young children although it can be something of a problem with the older child for whom the pragmatic disability may lead to extensive social inhibition. Thereafter decisions need to be made about the level selected and about whether strengths or weaknesses should be the target of the interventon. For example intact written language may be required in therapy. Clearly, social skills training may be one way in and this can be introduced using behavioural techniques. Modelling may be appropriate, but it is important that attention is paid to generalisation across different contexts. This is especially true in this client group, for whom meaning tends to be so context dependent.

Two clients are presented in the follwing chapters. Both described as having pragmatic disability. They are both able to produce reasonably well constructed sentences but both experience difficulties providing the appropriate level of information for their conversational partner, in essence in negotiating relevance. This leads to some similarities in the therapeutic strategies involved. However the two clients respond very differently to the treatment, leading the authors to postulate quite different explanations of their problems. The child, N, has more discrete problems, and his difficulties appear to resolve following a relatively short period of intervention. This leads Hampshire and Mogford-Bevan to maintain that the difficulties were indeed specific to pragmatic skills and thus opens the question as to how he managed to generalise prag-matic skills. By contrast the adult, RM, has persistent difficulties after an extensive period of treatment. It is this apparent resistance to focal treat-ment which leads Varley to suggest that his difficulties are part of a more central processing deficit.

Chapter 4.2
A case study of a child with pragmatic difficulties: assessment and intervention

AMANDA HAMPSHIRE AND KAY MOGFORD-BEVAN

Semantic–pragmatic disorder, first described by Rapin and Allen in 1983, became something of a buzz diagnosis in the 1980s. It seemed that suddenly there was a new group of communication disordered children whose difficulties had not really been discussed before. Speech and language therapists and educational psychologists immediately picked up on the diagnosis, and were able to apply it to a group of clients on their caseloads. However, the term was somewhat opaque to parents and teachers, as the disorder was difficult to describe precisely or to quantify. Most speech and language therapists continue to describe certain clients as having problems of a semantic or a pragmatic nature, and therapists seem to have a common understanding about what this diagnosis might mean, and of what they might do to help. In this paper, the details of a single case study of a child with pragmatic difficulties will be presented. It is hoped that the rigorous assessment procedure which is described here and which is based on linguistic analysis will help therapists to identify more clearly what is going wrong in the communication of other children who have pragmatic problems. The procedure provides baseline information which allows therapy to be focused and effective. The information is also accessible and can be shared with parents and teachers.

The linguistic information about the clusters of symptoms ascribed to pragmatic disorders has often been inadequate and too general to allow for differential diagnosis. It is generally agreed that children with pragmatic difficulties have fluent expressive language, but are unable to use it communicatively. They are unable to engage in meaningful interaction, and many of their utterances appear to be irrelevant. But there is no clear explanation as to why these children struggle to engage in conversation. Whether they fail to initiate or they fail to respond to verbal exchange, or only do so with certain conversational partners or in certain situations, is not clear. There are no criteria for irrelevancy in

194

conversation and conversational partners regularly cope with apparent non sequiturs, working together to make them relevant in the conversation. If this kind of difficulty is to be described accurately, then the sequential nature of conversation has to be taken into account, and the constant negotiation that takes place between speakers when they are talking needs to be considered. Obviously there is a need to collect language samples in a variety of different situations and with different conversational partners, in order to take into consideration the dynamic interaction between conversational partners. But without a detailed framework for analysis, the therapist will be unable to identify and quantify abnormal and recurring conversational strategies and behaviours in a systematic way. The principles of conversation analysis can be applied to data from naturally occurring language samples to address this problem. Conversation analysis investigates the principles and strategies used by participants in interaction. In this study, the procedure adopted draws heavily on the frameworks outlined by McTear (1985a, b) and Milroy (1988). This procedure allows the therapist to focus on specific aspects of the child's conversation, and to compare the child's conversational behaviours with the rules of conversation that have been observed in language normal speakers. It highlights for the therapist the rules of turn-taking and conversational exchange. It looks at mechanisms to repair breakdown in conversation and at the way meanings are conveyed in the complex relationship of form and function. It allows the therapist to look at conversational routines and the use of cohesion devices in the discourse. The therapist can then pinpoint and describe exactly why the child's conversation is disordered, and can begin to work directly on the abnormal conversational behaviours.

Given that previous descriptions of pragmatic difficulties have been rather subjective and have not been based on principled linguistic analysis, it has up to now been difficult to establish whether this is a specific and prescribed communication disorder, or whether pragmatic difficulties might be a symptom of another sort of disorder. There is a considerable body of evidence demonstrating that pragmatic difficulties often occur in consequence of receptive or expressive language difficulties. For example, language impaired children often experience difficulties in turn-taking, because they are unable to decode and encode messages quickly enough to participate in rapid verbal exchange. They tend to be less responsive in conversation, and may produce more unrelated responses than children with normal language, and they may be deficient in the range of speech acts they use (Brinton and Fujiki 1982, Fey and Leonard 1983, Craig and Evans 1989, McTear 1990). Language-impaired children may not be able to respond to requests for clarification adequately, because they do not have sufficient knowledge of alternate linguistic codings, and they are typically less likely than other children to request clarification (Gallagher and Darnton 1978, Donahue *et al.* 1980, Brinton and Fujiki 1982). On the other hand, problems with interaction could stem from a sociocognitive disorder such as autism or Asperger's syndrome. Autistic individuals tend to have profound semantic and pragmatic impairments (Tager-Flusberg 1981, Rapin 1987). Because of their inability to infer the beliefs of others, they are unable to use language for interactive purposes, and struggle to participate in conversation in spite of unimpaired phonological and grammatical development. If other diagnostic signs of autism are present, perhaps the pragmatic impairment should be seen as part of the disorder, rather than a syndrome in its own right. The use of a linguistic procedure to describe the conversational behaviours exhibited by the child could thus be vital in differential diagnosis. Once a standard procedure is used to analyse the conversational behaviours of different client groups, it is possible that patterns of behaviours will emerge allowing the therapist to distinguish between language-impaired and autistic children in a systematic rather than an intuitive way. It might also be possible to demonstrate that pragmatic problems can exist independently of any other communication or cognitive disorder.

Finally, although there has been some work carried out on the remediation of pragmatic difficulties in children (Conti-Ramsden and Gunn 1986, Jones *et al.* 1986, Hyde-Wright and Cray 1990), the efficacy of therapy has not been demonstrated empirically. The current climate in health intervention demands that therapists have a record of baseline functioning, and that they can demonstrate improvements in the areas that they have worked on. Unless intervention programmes that are designed to improve conversational skills are based on detailed linguistic analysis, it is difficult to measure outcome.

In this study, goals for intervention were selected on the basis of the linguistic analysis, and, following therapy, it was possible to demonstrate changes in the child's communication strategies, which had occurred as a result of intervention. Two different methods of treatment were compared in this study. In the first intervention phase of the study, behavioural methods of modelling, prompting and reinforcement were adopted. In the second intervention phase, a meta-linguistic approach was used in which the child was encouraged to discuss, practise and evaluate conversational rules. It was hoped that the child's response to the two different methods of treatment would indicate whether he had cognitive problems that could be responsible for his conversational disability. It was assumed that if the child had cognitive problems, he would not be able to learn to use the conversational rules he was taught in a flexible and creative way.

The subject

N was studied as a part of a research project designed to look at therapy in children with pragmatic difficulties. He was placed in a unit for children with speech and language problems at 5 years 9 months. Previous to this, he had spent a year in a school for autistic children, although a diagnosis of autism had never been made. N was studied over a period of 11 months. Following an initial assessment at 6 years 10 months, N was exposed to two blocks of therapy, each followed by reassessment, and a final assessment, when he was 7 years 9 months, after a period during which he received no treatment.

N was the youngest child of two teachers, and had twin siblings who were 4 years older than he was. His mother reported initially that there was no history of communication difficulties in the family, but she later mentioned that one of N's cousins had similar difficulties to N. N was born following a difficult pregnancy. His mother was admitted to hospital twice for bedrest as she had high blood pressure. She suffered influenza symptoms around the time of N's birth, for which she was treated with antibiotics. N was two weeks premature and there were no perinatal complications. N's mother noted that N's milestones occurred later than his those of siblings, especially in the area of speech and language development. However, he was walking at 11 months. There were no hearing or visual problems. N's parents became concerned about his development when he was approximately 18 months old. He was not using language to communicate and he exhibited some abnormal behaviours such as hand flapping and running around in circles.

From an early age, N exhibited some of the features that are considered to be diagnostic of autism. His mother reported that he clung to routine; for example, he was rigid in his eating habits, and became distressed if journeys out of the house involved taking a different route than usual. However, N's parents reported that he had built up relationships with the family members and was affectionate towards them from an early age. At 6 years 10 months N was still concerned with routine, particularly in relation to time. He would become upset if he was not able to do the usual thing at the usual time. N also exhibited some unusual preoccupations, which he would pursue to the exclusion of other activities. When interested in a topic, such as breeds of dog or a particular card or board game, N would persist in talking about it or playing it. Such preoccupations tended to be transitory, in that N would eventually lose interest in them and a new preoccupation would develop. N quickly established relationships with the adults in the language unit, but he rarely approached other children.

As with many language-impaired children, the development of N's symbolic play was noted to be delayed. Details from N's case notes indicated that his play was stereotypic and characterised by repetitive routines. However, he did participate in pretend play when guided by an adult. At 6 years 10 months N would copy the play of an adult or another child, by repeating their play schemes, often exactly, in similar situations. N liked formal rule-governed games like 'Yahtze'and 'Snakes and Ladders'.

N also had a history of significantly delayed language development. When first assessed by a speech and language therapist at 2 years 3 months, N was able to follow simple commands containing one information-carrying word, but had no meaningful speech. At 3 years 6 months, N had difficulties following verbal instructions unless they were accompanied by gesture and situational cues, and his expressive language was characterised by echolalia and learned phrases. At 6 years 10 months N was scoring at a low average level in standard assessments of his understanding. For example he achieved a score on the 25th centile in the Test for the Reception of Grammar (Bishop 1982). In this assessment, N demonstrated that he could understand quite complex grammatical forms, including sentences containing embedded clauses, and complex negatives. However, he frequently answered only three out of the four stimuli correctly, and therefore had to be marked as failing the block testing that particular sentence structure. At 6 years 10 months he was able to use the appropriate grammatical structures to ask questions, give commands and make statements or denials, and was linking sentences using the processes of coordination and subordination. He was also using past tense forms correctly. Problems with velar sounds noted at 5 years 8 months had resolved, but the rhythm and intonation of N's speech was observed to be atypical.

Assessment based on conversation analysis

As might have been predicted, information from the routine clinical assessments gave little insight into the nature of N's difficulties, and no indications at all about how to help him. Such assessments stripped away the variations of topic, context and conversational partner which appeared to be precisely the features that N found difficult. N's difficulties needed to be assessed in those settings where he was experiencing problems. An assessment framework was therefore designed following the principles of conversation analysis.

Data were collected from two sources in the school setting.

• N was video recorded playing with three different conversational partners. These included the nursery nurse in the language unit (referred to as A). N knew the nursery nurse very well, having worked with her over the previous year. N was also recorded playing with familiar and unfamiliar children. The familiar children (referred to as FC1 and FC2) were also in the language unit in the same academic year as N. They had both had severe phonological disorders which had resolved with therapy. The unfamiliar child (referred to as UC) was in the mainstream class where N was integrated, and was also in the same academic year group. Video sessions lasted approximately

20 minutes, and N and his partner were left to play with a variety of toys (e.g. play people camper, fire engine and spaceship, Lego etc.).

• N was observed in a variety of different settings in school. Paper and pencil notes were made in each setting detailing the identity of N's conversational partners, the context, the topic of conversation and the linguistic forms used to initiate and respond. N was observed in the language unit classroom, where he was familiar with both the routine and the children and staff. He was also observed in the mainstream classroom, where he integrated for one day a week with his mainstream peers. He was observed in the yard at playtimes, and in the dining hall at lunchtimes.

A multiple-baseline across behaviours design was adopted, focusing on seven independent conversational behaviours.

Initiations

These were defined as utterances where N attempted to start a conversation. The linguistic form of N's initiations was examined and an evaluation was made as to whether his initiations weakly or strongly demanded a response from the addressee. It was also noted whether N's initiations related to his own previous utterances and his own activities, or whether he showed an interest in the topics of conversation and activities introduced by others.

Directives

The linguistic form of N's directives was noted to see what form he used to direct others. Whether he was able to change the form of his directives according to the addressee and the situation was also considered.

Attention getting devices

It was noted whether N understood the use of attention getting devices. Whether he was able to signal to a potential addressee that he was speaking or was going to speak to them was considered. It was also noted whether N appreciated the necessity of following up the summons implication of an attention getting device with a reason for the summons.

Social routines

N's use of greetings and partings and his use of politeness words and sequences were noted.

Responses

N's awareness of his obligations in conversation was assessed. It was noted whether he was able to fulfil his obligations in conversation by responding to the initiations of others. Whether he could relate his responses to the preceding utterance of his conversational partner was also considered, and whether he could share in the responsibility of maintaining a topic over several turns.

Repair and clarification

The data were scanned to see if N requested clarification in situations where he did not understand and if he was able to revise his own utterances in response to requests for clarification from his conversational partners. N's strategies for renegotiating conversation when his conversational partner failed to reply to his initiations were also examined.

Cohesion

Devices used by N to maintain and link discourse were noted.

Profile of conversational behaviours

N's conversational behaviours are described in this section. Transcripts from the video assessment are presented below (Table 4.2.1) and will be referred to in order to illustrate specific conversational behaviours.

Initiations

N often tried to start up a conversation using a form that did not demand a response from the addressee. The majority of N's utterances were declarative in form, and there was therefore no obligation for his conversational partner to reply. N usually commented on what he was doing, or on what was happening around him rather than trying to engage the other person in a topic that might have been mutually interesting. N showed very little interest in the activities of other children and rarely commented on what they were doing or what they had said. This is reflected in Table 4.2.1 where, despite repeated attempts by FC1 to get N to join in the play sequence (lines 25–26, 31, 50, 52), N's utterances relate only to putting the play people either on a bike or in the car. The responsibility therefore of maintaining the interaction fell to N's conversational partner, who had to take up N's choice of topic. Adults were typically very good at identifying when N was trying to start up a conversation, but other children frequently failed to respond to N's declarative utterances. This inability to take account of the utterances of others has implications for cohesive structure of the discourse.

Table 4.2.1 Transcript 1

1	FC1:	*ah you've broke the motorbike*	(N tries to put a man on a bike)
2		*no you haven't*	
3		*_ I can fix it*	
4		*_ _ N, fixed the motorbike for you*	(FC1 fixes another man on a bike)
5	N:	*mhm*	
6	FC1:	*I think it's better if you ride the car*	
7		*_ do you?*	
8	N:	*_ _ yeah*	(N continues to try to fix his man on the bike)
9		*I better ride this bike on#*	
10	FC1:	*_ _ _ _ _ _ _ _ ee*	(FC1 takes a motorbike rider out of the car)
11		*_ _ _ _ _ _ _ ee look what I've got*	
12		*I've got a man with a motorbike suit*	
13		*he's a proper motorbike rider*	
14		*_ _ _ oh*	
15	N:	*_ _ got that arm on*	(N continues to try to put man on bike)
16	FC1:	*_ _ _ I'm fixed*	
17		*I'm fixed*	
18		*_ _ (symbolic noise)*	
19		*wait for me brother*	(FC1 puts two men on motorbike)
20		*get on brother*	
21	N:	*_ want help to get on*	
22		*_ I need help to get on this bike*	(N continues to try to put man on bike and holds bike towards FC1)
23		*_ this bike turns corners all the time*	
24	FC1:	*(symbolic noise)*	(FC1 drives motorbike up in the air)
25		*you said how did you do that*	
26		*_ go on*	(N continues to try to put man on bike)
27		*_ (symbolic noise)*	
28		*I'm getting on mate bye*	
29		*(symbolic noise)*	
30		*I'm going on my cycle*	
31		*_ oh where's your cycle?*	(FC1 plays with play people)
32		*_ you had two cycles*	
33		*one's#*	
34		*I know two cycles*	
35		*but I'm going on this cycle*	(N continues to try to put man on bike)
36		*_ motorcycle yes*	
37		*easy buy it*	
38		*drive it*	
39		*buy it and drive it*	
40		*_ biker go*	
41		*_ _ _ (symbolic noise)*	

(contd)

Table 4.2.1 (contd)

42	N:	_ *different car*	(N gives up and puts toys back in basket)
43	FC1:	(symbolic noise)	
44		*bye*	
45		*see you tomorrow*	
46	N:	_ *we're all going in my car*	(N starts to put men in car)
47	FC1:	*bye*	
48	N:	*I'm getting full*	
49		_ *I'm getting full*	
50	FC1:	_ *we're on holiday aren't we N*	
51		_ _ *right*	
52		*N we're on holiday now*	
53	N:	*and all the rest#*	(N gets more men from basket and moves them towards FC1's camper)
54		*and all the rest can go in your car*	
55	FC1:	*a barbie*	(FC1 finds a barbecue)
56		_ _ *right we on holiday now aren't we N*	

Transcription conventions
1. Pauses are marked by _ or a sequence of _. Each _ is equivalent to one pulse of the speaker's rhythm.
2. Non-verbal responses and other remarks which put the utterances into context and are relevant to their interpretation are written in brackets next to the utterances with which they co-occurred.
3. Unfinished utterances are marked by # at the point where the speaker stopped talking.
4. Utterances are referred to in the text by the transcript number in which they occurred and a line reference. Where there are instances of several utterances which illustrate the same conversational behaviour, all those utterances are cited in the text.

Directives

N frequently used declarative forms to direct others, and, as a result, many of his attempts to direct others were unsuccessful, because his directives were not recognised as such. In Table 4.2.1, N's non-verbal behaviour, looking pleadingly at FC1 and holding out the bike and the play person to him, indicated that N wanted FC1 to help put the person on the bike (lines 21–23). FC1 evidently does not recognise this as an implicit request. Table 4.2.2 records some of the directives/requests that N used in the observation assessment. Often only the non-verbal context in which these utterances occurred indicated what N wanted. For example, when N was struggling to open his crisps, he might have been merely commenting that he could not open them, in which case his statement would have been appropriate, but his non-verbal behaviour (struggling with the packet and then holding it out to the adult) suggested that he was requesting help. The use of a declarative to request help is not unusual, particularly in young children, but N's apparent inability to change the form of his directive so that his meaning became more explicit is. On only two occasions was N observed to change the form of his directive into a more recognisable request, e.g. a polar interrogative. It was interesting that adults generally recognised N's declarative requests, interpreting what he wanted and complying, but other children did not. Other children did respond, however, on the few occasions when N used a polar interrogative form.

Table 4.2.2 Examples of N's directive in the initial observation assessment

Transcript	Context
I done good work	In both cases N was standing next to the class
I think I did very well	teacher. He had finished his work and evidently wanted it marked
I need to spell Margaret	N was standing next to the class teacher and evidently needed a spelling to complete his work
I got a poppy	N was standing in front of the speech and language therapist holding a poppy and trying to get it into his jumper
I can't open this	N was standing in front of an adult trying to open a packet of crisps

Attention getting devices

N did not appear to appreciate that attention getting devices should occur as a three-part sequence: a summons, a response, and a reason for the summons. Frequently, N did not use any attention getting device at all to alert the listener to attend to his subsequent utterance. Consequently potential addressees were not aware that they were being addressed, and did not respond to his initiations. On other occasions, N used an attention getting device, often another child's name, without following it up with a reason for the summons when the child responded. Typically he would repeat the child's name several times, but did not fulfil his conversational obligation to provide the third part of the sequence. N was also observed to use gaze to attract attention and was often noted to stare intently at a potential addressee before speaking to them.

Social routines

There were no occasions where N was observed to initiate a greeting or parting sequence during either the video or the observation assessment. Lines 44–47 in Table 4.2.1 demonstrate that N was also unlikely to respond to such exchanges. Neither did N use politeness routines. For example he would push past people if they were in his way and did not say 'excuse me'. Nor did he use words such as 'please' and 'thank you'.

Responses

N characteristically presented with difficulties in fulfilling his conversational obligation to fill the response slots set up for him by his conversational partners. He often appeared to be unaware of the utterances of his conversational partner, and he failed to respond at all. This is reflected in the high percentage of nil responses, particularly to the initiations of other children (Table 4.2.3) and in lines 31, 50 and 52 of Transcript 1 (Table 4.2.1). FC1 had to repeat and rephrase his utterances in order to try to elicit a response from N. N could not even reply when he was told explicitly what to say (lines 25–26). On other occasions, N apparently recognised his obligation to reply, and he filled the response slot, but he demonstrated that he did not appreciate the tendency of conversation to be organised in closely related paired turns. Schegloff and Sacks (1973) describe these as **adjacency pairs**, where the first part of the pair sets up expectations about the second part of the pair. N frequently failed to meet the expectations of his conversational partner by contributing an utterance (the second part of the pair) that did not correspond with his partner's utterance (the first part of the pair). Sometimes, it was clear that although N had said the right thing he had not really taken account of what the other person had said (see lines 6–8 of Transcript 1).

Table 4.2.3 The percentage number of adult and other child initiations to which N failed to respond in the initial and final observation assessments

| | Percentage of nil responses | |
	to the initiations of adults	to the initiations of other children
Initial observation assessment	11	50
Final observation assessment	10	14

Because of their ability to take account of N's difficulties, adults were much better at maintaining conversation with N. For example, in the video session with N, the nursery nurse accepted and responded to N's initiations and tried to build on them to maintain the conversation. She repeated and rephrased her initiations until she received a satisfactory response. She often set up N's responses in question–answer sequences, helping him to reply appropriately by giving him a forced alternative or a phonemic cue. Other children lacked the conversational skills to compensate for N's difficulties in this way. For example, in Transcript 1, although FC1 is aware of N's failure to fill the response slot about the play people going on holiday, his device of repeating N's name (lines 50, 52, 56) to try to get N to agree does not work. He was also less able to follow up N's initiations as topics of conversation and could not structure the conversation to ensure N would respond. Again this has implications for the cohesive nature of discourse. When N was with other children, no shared topic emerged, and an interactive discourse could not develop. Unless the conversation was specifically structured to accommodate N's conversational problems, conversation became less of a dialogue and more like two concurrent monologues.

Repair and clarification

N was not observed to request clarification on any occasion, even when it was evident that he had not understood what the speaker had said. For example, the teacher in the mainstream class had been teaching the children French in N's absence. When she said 'asseyez-vous' all the other children sat down. N, however, did not respond to this command, either by taking steps to find out what she meant, or by copying the other children.

N did recognise the need to respond to requests for clarification but relied heavily on non-verbal means and on repetition to resolve mishearings or misunderstandings. These strategies were not always very successful. In the example in Table 4.2.4, N and UC were looking at a doll's house in which there was an ordinary wall clock. N commented that the clock said four o'clock, and then went on to explain how this would appear on a digital clock on a television. UC clearly did not understand what N was talking about, but N was not able to clarify himself. N clearly recognised that he had not been understood, and realised that he needed to do something about it, but if non-verbal means (pointing) or repetition failed to clarify the situation, he could not mobilise other strategies.

Table 4.2.4 Transcript 2

N: _ _ _ _ *that says four o'clock on there* (points to clock)
UC: *where?*
       four o'clock on where?
N: *there* (points to clock again)
       _that says oh oh
UC: *four o'clock?*
N: *on the television clock*
       the two ohs mean o'clock
UC: *pardon*
N: *the two ohs mean o'clock on the television clock*
UC: *how did you know?*
N: *because the two ohs mean o'clock*
UC: *mhm right*
       _ _ very good N

N also relied on repetition to re-initiate on occasions when his partner failed to respond to him. He used repetition as a means of demanding his partner's attention and eliciting a reply. He continued to repeat himself until the other person replied. N did not seem to be aware of the other strategies he could use to elicit a response (e.g. using an attention getting device or changing the form of his utterance so that it more strongly demanded a response from the addressee).

Cohesion

N's inability to respond to the contributions of his conversational partner has obvious implications for the cohesive structure of the discourse. N was not able to follow up topics of conversation over several turns unless the conversation was carefully structured for him. His utterances did, however, have some internal consistency, as Transcript 1 demonstrates.

N often repeated all or part of his conversational partner's utterance, as a means of agreeing with his partner, or of affirming what his partner had just said. Often an elliptical response or a yes/no response would have been more usual. For example, here N confirmed that his car was not driving to Beamish:

N: *this car's not going*
A: *it's not going?*
N: *it's not going*

This strategy was only noted when N was conversing with an adult.

Therapy

The initial assessment pinpointed several areas where N was experiencing difficulties, and also to some extent explained why he was having problems in conversation. Therapy procedures were designed to address these difficulties. The two different intervention methods were each continued over a period of one term. N was reassessed using the same procedure after each block of therapy and then after a three month period of no treatment.

Intervention I

A behavioural approach was adopted in the first intervention phase of the study. N's difficulties with directives and with attention getting devices were considered to be particularly significant, not only because these are early functions to develop (Halliday 1975), but also because N's failure to appreciate the rules of securing attention and making requests rendered so many of his interactions unsuccessful. N was taught to use the polar interrogative form to direct others. This form was felt to be polite enough to be acceptable with most addressees, whatever their relationship with N, and in most situations. N was also taught to use the word *please*, as this would immediately mark his utterance as a directive, and also make it more polite and therefore more acceptable to the addressee. In addition, N was encouraged to use the name of the addressee as part of his directive. This would make it obvious who was being addressed, and would direct that person's attention to the subsequent polar interrogative.

N was seen for five sessions on his own in the speech and language therapy room. Activities were set up where N could not complete a task unless he asked the therapist to perform some action. For example, N was asked to complete several jigsaw puzzles, but was not given all the pieces. N had to ask the therapist for the missing pieces. The target structure, a polar interrogative, was modelled for N to imitate:

> If you want the penguin piece, N, you could ask. You could say:
> *Miss W please can I have the penguin*

When N imitated the directive correctly, he was rewarded with whatever he had asked for, and told that he had done '*good asking*'. If he failed to imitate a directive, it was modelled again until he did repeat it. Once N was confidently imitating directives, the therapist started to prompt him rather than model the directive:

> If you want the penguin, N, you will have to ask   .

Prompts were gradually faded as N began to identify for himself when he needed to make a request. Activities were then set up in the language unit classroom, and N was encouraged to address his directives to the other children and the other members of staff . Directives were once again modelled and prompted, and N was rewarded when he made a request. N was then encouraged to make requests in naturally occurring classroom activities, both in the language unit and in the mainstream classroom where he integrated for one afternoon a week. The staff in the language unit and N's parents were encouraged to model and prompt N's directives. Whenever N made a request spontaneously, it was reinforced by complying with the request and by telling N that he had done '*good asking*'.

N responded very well to this approach, and started to use directives in a variety of different situations. He began to develop some flexibility in that if a declarative used as a request did not meet with the response he expected, N would change the form of his directive to a polar interrogative so that the other person would comply. He also began to use attention getting devices and *please* with other utterances, not just with directives. In addition, in the observation reassessment following this block of therapy, the percentage number of occasions where N failed to respond to the initiations of other children had decreased from 50% to 29%.

Intervention II

A meta-linguistic approach was adopted in Intervention II. N worked as a member of a group in with the other children in the language unit. The group observed the class teacher and the therapist modelling target communication behaviours and the children practised these within the group setting. They also observed role plays of poor communication, and were encouraged to discuss why communication had broken down in these sequences. The children monitored and evaluated one another's communication skills within the group and were also actively encouraged to use the skills as relevant situations arose in the course of the school day. The group sessions took place three to four times a week for one term. N's family were kept informed of the aims of the group, and were asked to discuss and practise good communication skills with N at home.

Intervention II focused mainly on N's ability to respond to the non-verbal and verbal initiations of others. In particular N and the other children in the group were encouraged to initiate and respond to greeting and parting sequences. They were made aware of various greeting and parting sequences, and rehearsed using them in the context of the group. They were also encouraged to identify the situations in which such sequences would normally occur and prompted to use them in these situations. The children were also made aware of the strategies they could use to attract the attention of an addressee who failed to respond to greetings/partings (e.g. tap the other person, say the greeting more loudly, move nearer to the other person, etc.). The children were taught to watch one another's faces and to identify when someone smiled at them. They were encouraged to smile back. The children watched role plays of 'good' and 'bad' listening, and were encouraged to distinguish between the two. They then thought of some rules for 'good listening' which involved non-verbal behaviours (e.g. sitting still, looking at the speaker, etc.), and verbal behaviours (e.g. using backchannel words and phrases, asking topic related questions, etc.). Everyone in the group practised 'good listening', and evaluated one another's listening skills. The children were also encouraged to consider how to initiate a repair sequence when an addressee failed to respond to them, or when they had not heard/understood what had been said to them.

Reassessment: the profile of conversational behaviours following therapy

N's conversational strategies were reassessed following therapy, and after a period of no treatment. As in the first assessment all aspects of N's conversation were examined, and significant changes were observed in those areas that had been targeted in therapy.

Initiations

Transcripts 3 and 4 demonstrate that N's initiations demanded a response much more strongly than had been the case before therapy. N no longer relied on declarative utterances, but used attention getting devices, questions and imperatives in a much more meaningful way to focus the attention of his conversational partners, to give commands and to ask for information (Table 4.2.5, Transcript 3, lines 1, 2, 6, 24; Transcript 4, lines 2, 33). In using these more forceful forms, N set up an obligation such that his conversational partners were required to respond to his utterances and to comply with his instructions. Moreover, N's initiations indicate that he had started to take an interest in the topics of conversation introduced by his partners and in their play activities. N's initiations were no longer restricted to his own train of thought, but were, on the contrary, actively related to shared topics, activities and interests.

Directives

Table 4.2.6 demonstrates the contrast in the linguistic form of N's directives prior to therapy with those occurring following therapy. This is also reflected in Transcript 3 (line 2) where N used an imperative to tell FC2 to put somebody on the bike. N's directives were much more explicit and therefore more readily identifiable to his conversational partners. Other children in particular were much more likely to comply.

N also began to show an understanding of the underlying rules of directing and requesting. For example, he would use the polar interrogative form as he had been taught when interacting with adults or less familiar children, but when playing with the familiar children from the language unit, he tended to use imperative forms. This demonstrates a sensitivity to the familiarity and status of the addressee that had not been taught in therapy. N also began to demonstrate a flexibility in his communication strategies that had been notably lacking in the first assessment. When he did not get the response he expected/wanted, he would change the form of his directive in order to get what he wanted. For example, here N required a rubber, and spontaneously asked another child for theirs:

> N:*I need a rubber*
> *Please Andrew can I borrow your rubber?*

Table 4.2.5 Transcripts 3 and 4

Transcript 3

1	N:	*it hasn't got somebody on it Paul*	(N points to bike)
2		*put somebody on it*	(N gives FC2 a man)
3		*a girl or a boy*	
4		*or a lady or a man*	(FC2 discards man)
5		_ _ *put the one with#*	(N passes him another man)
6		*look*	(N finds a helmet)
7		*look at that*	
8		_ _ *this is a helmet*	(N gives helmet to FC2)
9		*has to have a helmet on first*	
10		*so he doesn't fall off*	(N drives car across table)
11	FC2:	_ _ *it's another motorbike ride*	(FC2 finds a motorbike which
12		_ _ (symbolic noise)	already has a man on and drives it)
13	N:	*just a minute*	
14		*you have to go through here*	(N drives car between two piles of toys)
15		*I've got a little maze*	
16		*I've got a maze for you*	
17		*I've got a maze*	
18		*we could put these things there and these things there*	
19		*so you can go through the middle*	(N drives the car between the two piles)
20		_ _ (sings)	
21	FC2:	(symbolic noise)	(FC2 drives his motorbike between
22		*beep beep*	the two piles of toys)
23		(symbolic noise)	
24	N:	*lets make a new maze*	(N moves the two piles of toys)
25		*we're going to put this side at this side*	
26		_ _ (sings)	
27		_ _ *last couple goes in there*	(N puts two toys in car)
28	FC2:	(unintelligible)	
29	N:	(sings)	
30	FC2:	(sings)	
31		(unintelligible)	
32		(symbolic noise)	
33	N:	*the camper squeaks when it goes round corners#*	
34		*the camper squeaks*	(N drives car round table)
35	FC2:	(symbolic noise)	(FC2 drives motorbike)
36		_ *move*	
37		(symbolic noise)	
38	N:	*it's stopping for one minute*	(N stops car)
39	FC2:	(symbolic noise)	
40		*hey can me have the car?*	(FC2 takes hold of N's car)
41	N:	*and I'll have the camper*	
42		(unintelligible)	
43	FC2:	*wait here*	(N and FC2 exchange toys)

Table 4.2.5 (contd)

Transcript 4

1	UC:	*could you find some fourers?*	(UC builds Lego model)
2	N:	*what's fourers like?*	
3	UC:	*like _ these*	(UC finds fourer and shows N)
4		*one two three four*	
5	N:	*_ no*	(N rakes through Lego pieces and discards them)
6		*that#*	
7		(unintelligible) *not that can't be*	(N finds and offers a fourer)
8	UC:	*that is the kind but I don't want that on*	
9		*it has to be red*	
10	N:	*and it has to be red*	
11		*I wonder* (unintelligible)	(N rakes through Lego pieces)
12		*I found sixers*	
13	UC:	*sixers*	
14		*that's a three-er*	(UC rakes through Lego pieces)
15	N:	*that's a three*	
16		(sings)	
17	UC:	*found some more*	
18		(unintelligible)	
19	N:	*I found two fourers that are red*	
20	UC:	*let me see yours*	(N holds fourers out)
21		*oh good*	(UC takes them)
22		*_ _ _ thank you very much*	
23		*_ (sings)*	
24	N:	*that's#*	
25	UC:	(sings)	
26	N:	*I can't find#*	
27		*_ _ _ _ I've found a#*	(N hands Lego piece to UC)
28	UC:	*_ _ _ exactly what I need*	
29	N:	*_ _ _ and I found another fourer*	(N finds another Lego piece)

Attention getting devices

Table 4.2.6 and Transcript 3 (line 1) demonstrate that N began to use vocatives consistently to secure the attention of the addressee when he spoke to them. N started to use vocatives as attention getting devices with a range of different utterance types, and not just directives/requests. He also started to use other attention getting devices e.g. notice verbs like *look* and *watch*, topic opening phrases and non-verbal cues (Transcript 3, lines 6–7, 13).

Social routines

N spontaneously began to initiate and respond to greeting and parting sequences, particularly when he arrived at or left school. He would greet people during the course of the school day when he met them. He also showed that he was aware of the therapist when she was observing him, and would smile and wave at her, where he had seemed oblivious to her in the first assessment.

Table 4.2.6 Examples of N's directives in subsequent assessments

Transcript	Context
Mrs B would you try and fix this one	N asked nursery teacher to put the roof on the camper van
Miss D please can I have some paper	N asked class teacher to give him some paper
Can I have that one?	N addressed dinner lady to indicate what he wanted for lunch
Please Miss W would you mark my work?	N asked speech and language therapist to mark his work
Lisa can I borrow your rubber?	N asked child in mainstream class for a rubber
Will someone please sharpen it?	N asked a group of children in mainstream class if one of them would sharpen his pencil
Stuart don't push me	N asked a language unit child not to push him in the dinner queue
Get in the back Sally please	N asked language unit child to get in the back of his imaginary car
Lets go and chase each other	N asked a language unit child to play chase with him at playtime.

N regularly used *please* with his imperative and his polar interrogative directives. He started to use other politeness words as well, such as *excuse me* and *sorry*. For example, he apologised to the therapist for stepping on her toe.

Responses

Transcripts 3 and 4 demonstrate that N was much more aware of the need to respond in conversation. FC2 and UC do not need to repeat or revise their utterances in order to get a response from N. Following intervention, N recognised his obligation to fill the response slots set up for him (Transcript 3, lines 40–41; transcript 4, lines 1–2, 9–10). He also provided responses that met with the expectations of his conversational partners. There was consequently a real sense of interaction and shared topic which had been lacking in the first assessment. Table 4.2.3 illustrates the dramatic decrease in the percentage of nil responses to the initiations of the children with whom N was observed.

It was interesting to note how the behaviour of other children towards N began to change. The initial assessment had indicated a big discrepancy between N's response to adults and his response to other children. It also revealed that other children tended to ignore N and were unlikely to initiate interaction with him. However during intervention, this began to change. Other children were quick to react to his directives or requests, and even began to offer objects and assistance to him. At this stage, it was not clear whether this was the result of N's new communication strategies, or was a feature dependent upon the presence of the therapist. However this change was maintained after Intervention I had been completed, during Intervention II when the therapist assumed a less obtrusive role and in the subsequent reassessment phases of the study. In the final assessment, the number of occasions where N was approached by other children had more than doubled. It is argued that N's new responsiveness to others made communication with him more rewarding and therefore other children were more likely to interact with him. That N was no longer socially isolated was perhaps one of the most significant results of therapy.

Repair and clarification

Line 2 in Transcript 4 demonstrates that N had learned to seek clarification in an active way and could feed back to his conversational partner when he had not understood what they meant. On occasion, N asked for more information (as here) but on other occasions N would use words like *what* in order to ask for clarification. N continued to rely on repetition when responding to a request for clarification from his conversational partner and to re-initiate a failed interaction. However, he did begin to demonstrate the flexibility to alter his utterances to make his intentions more explicit to the addressee, and to elicit a response. N also began to use attention getting devices to call the addressee's attention to utterances which they had ignored.

Cohesion

The improvement in N's ability to respond on topic and to maintain topic over several turns had an obvious impact on the cohesive structure of the discourse which is evident in Transcripts 3 and 4. N continued to repeat all or part of his conversational partner's utterance to acknowledge what they had said. As before, this only occurred when N was interacting with an adult.

Outcomes and discussion

The evidence of the study was that intervention was effective. N's communication improved considerably following intervention, and reassessment after a period of no treatment indicated that N had retained what he had learned. It is of course possible that the changes that took place in N's communication behaviours were not related to the therapy. The design of the study does not preclude the possibility of spontaneous improvement over time. In the natural course of development, it would be predicted that changes would have taken place in N's communication behaviours, and good clinical practice demanded that intervention goals focused on behaviours that were already emerging. It can only be argued that N's communication had been closely monitored over the 18 months prior to this study, and he had changed relatively little during that period. It is also difficult to demonstrate that the intervention programmes designed to change specific behaviours were directly responsible for changes in those behaviours. The multiple baseline across behaviours design implies that the conversational behaviours assessed and treated were independent of one another. It is suggested that the conversational behaviours were in fact interrelated, and that intervention focusing on one behaviour was very likely to have effects on the others. This was borne out following the first intervention phase, where it was clear that the changes in N's requesting behaviour had implications for his ability to respond in conversation. On the other hand, it cannot be disputed that there were changes in N's requesting behaviour following Intervention I, and changes in his responding behaviour following Intervention II.

The findings of this study strongly support the hypothesis that pragmatic disability can exist in isolation. N's difficulties in conversation could not be attributed to a grammatical disorder, in spite of his history of delayed language development. The initial assessment demonstrated that N did not lack the grammatical competence to formulate polar interrogative sentences. On the contrary, he just did not use them in situations where they would normally occur. Moreover, he had no difficulties acquiring the polar interrogative form, and using it in a flexible and creative way with a variety of different auxiliary verbs. This presumably would not have been possible if N had had a grammatical impairment. Similarly the evidence of intervention strongly suggested that N's problems were not of an autistic nature either. Recent research suggests that the features of autism are best explained by the child's inability to infer the mental states of others (Baron-Cohen *et al.* 1989). Autistic children are said to be unable to 'mentalise', and cannot think or reason about the content of their own or other people's minds. N, on the contrary, was interested in what other people were thinking and started to use language purposefully to achieve interactive ends, sharing topics introduced by his conversational partners, and actively trying to find out more about what the other person knew or felt. He began to use language creatively in imaginative and pretend play. He adapted his requests according to the status of the addressee, and he anticipated when listeners might have difficulty understanding him, modifying his utterances in order to make his meaning clearer. Furthermore, although no theory of mind tasks were carried out formally with N as part of this study, the week after the final reassessment N shared a joke with the nursery nurse in the language unit which required knowledge of a shared experience some days previously. N referred back to this shared experience in a different context, knowing that the nursery nurse would appreciate what he meant. These features indicate that N was able to take account of the contents of other people's minds. The other significant feature which strongly suggested that N was not autistic was his ability to learn. Prizant and Schuler (1987) argue that autistic individuals process information in an inflexible way, memorising ideas and patterns as a whole. N, in contrast, demonstrated a more analytical style of learning, and was apparently able to appreciate the underlying rules. For example, he extended his new conversational strategies beyond the situations and addressees to which he had been exposed in therapy. He was able to extract the meaning behind the use of directives and started to change their form according to the addressee and the situation. This presumably would not have occurred had N been autistic.

In fact, many of the conversational features that N exhibited have been noted in much younger children who are developing language normally. For example, many young children use declarative or 'need statements' to direct others (Ervin-Tripp 1977). Young children also tend to use declaratives to initiate interaction (Craig and Gallagher 1979). The use of gaze, the repetition of vocatives and the use of questions have all been noted as attention getting strategies employed by children in the early stages of language development (Keenan and Schieffelin 1976, Atkinson 1979). Young children also tend to be so involved in their own activities that they ignore the conversational contributions of others and do not reply. In N's case, where assessment and therapy eliminated the diagnoses of grammatical and autistic impairments, N's conversational behaviours could be described as being severely delayed. It would be theoretically elegant to suggest that, like phonological and grammatical disorders, pragmatic disorders may represent a severe delay in pragmatic development, and may be characterised by pragmatic features typical of a much less mature population.

The evidence suggests that N's conversational behaviours are not atypical of pragmatic disorder. Many of the features noted as abnormal in N's communication have been documented elsewhere in the literature describing children with pragmatic disorders. Willcox and Mogford-Bevan (1995b) describe another child, Daniel, who exhibited a very similar conversational profile to N. Conti-Ramsden and Gunn (1986) noted that the child they studied was late to use requests, and Greenlee (1981) observed that her subject used declaratives with directive force in the same way as N did. Often children with pragmatic disorders fail to use any strategies at all to gain the attention of their conversational partner (Blank *et al.* 1979) or they use unusual means to solicit attention and to initiate interaction e.g. asking questions to which they already know the answer or to which their conversational partner cannot know the answer (Greenlee 1981, Bishop and Adams 1989). Like N, children with pragmatic disorders find it difficult to share the responsibility of maintaining cohesive discourse. They find it difficult to respond on topic, or to maintain topic over several turns. Often they offer no response at all, or their reply does not relate to the preceding utterance of their conversational partner (Greenlee 1981; Conti-Ramsden and Gunn 1986, Jones *et al.* 1986). Both Bishop and Adams (1989) and Greenlee (1981) also report that the children are unable to provide adequate responses to requests for clarification. Blank and her colleagues found that, like N, the child they studied repeated his utterances when his initiations were ignored until he received a response. Obviously there is a need for much more research to establish to what extent these findings would hold true for other subjects. More exciting is the possibility that different groups of children might present with different clusters of conversational behaviours, thus enabling the speech and language therapist to contribute in the differential diagnosis of, for example, autism and language disorder, in an objective and scientific way.

The benefits of conversational analysis in the assessment and treatment of adults with communication disorders are also being identified and explored (Lesser and Milroy 1993, Perkins *et al.* 1995, Wilkinson 1995). It is interesting that there are many similarities in the conversational features exhibited by pragmatically impaired children and dysphasic adults, not least of which is their dependence on their conversational partner. Because of their linguistic difficulties, dysphasic adults often rely heavily on their conversational partners to interpret what they are trying to say, and to structure conversation for them. They often rely on others to anticipate trouble spots in the conversation, and to take responsibility for conversation repair. As with children with pragmatic difficulties, conversations with dysphasic adults are often difficult to disentangle, and clarification and repair take place over many utterances rather than over two or three as is the case with language normal speakers. Dysphasic adults also tend to use abnormal or idiosyncratic conversational strategies. For example, they may use hand movements or body posture to help maintain their turn in conversation, and to avoid interruption. Conversational analysis enables the therapist to identify these features, and tackle them directly in cases where they are affecting communication adversely. Interaction may be facilitated by raising the awareness of the client and of their families about the different strategies that are being used, and by alerting them as to where problems are most likely to occur.

Conclusion

Ultimately, the success of therapy has to be assessed not in terms of formal tests, but in terms of an improvement in spontaneous communication. Conversation analysis provides a practical framework for assessing real life and real time communication in a measurable way. In N's case, conversation analysis enabled the therapist to identify and explain why N was unable to participate successfully in conversation. It provided information about more usual conversation strategies, and thus enabled the therapist to teach N how to converse in a more normal way. The change that took place in N's communication speaks for itself.

Acknowledgements

We would like to thank N's family, and the staff at his school. We are also grateful to North Durham Community Health Care Trust for facilitating this research.

Some of the material discussed here has already appeared in Willcox and Mogford-Bevan (1995b).

Chapter 4.3
The treatment of communication deficits following right hemisphere lesion

ROSEMARY VARLEY

The role of the left hemisphere of the cerebral cortex in the mediation of language behaviour was recognised in the middle of the nineteenth century (Broca 1865). Lesions to the left, language-dominant cortex often result in aphasia, with very obvious impairments of grammar and lexis. Lesions to the right hemisphere (RH), in contrast, often result in complex visuospatial disruptions, for example, visual agnosia, constructional apraxia, and neglect. Communicative impairments following right, non-language-dominant hemisphere lesion were first described by Eisenson (1962). These impairments were more subtle and qualitatively different to the difficulties in language comprehension, lexical retrieval and grammatical structure of aphasic language.

Since Eisenson's initial observations, the right hemisphere 'syndrome' has been expanded and now includes the following characteristics:

- **non-verbal communication** – paucity of facial expression and abnormalities of eye contact (Borod *et al.* 1986)
- **prosody** – difficulties in both the encoding and decoding of emotional prosodic information (Heilman *et al.* 1975, Ross and Mesulam 1979) and linguistic stress (Bryan 1989)
- **lexicon** – semantic errors in lexical comprehension tasks (e.g. Lesser 1974, Gainotti *et al.* 1983), and errors in picture naming
- **non-literal language** – literal interpretation of metaphors, difficulties going beyond given information to make inferences, difficulties in the interpretation of jokes (Brownell *et al.* 1983, Myers 1994, Winner and Gardner 1977)
- **conversation and discourse** – abnormally long talk turns, sudden unsignalled topic changes, and excessive, verbose language (Joanette *et al.* 1986, Sherratt and Penn 1990).

Certain of these characteristics are predictable from what is known about right hemisphere information processing abilities. The right hemisphere has been shown to have a role in face processing (Young and Ratcliffe 1983), dealing with emotional information (Bear 1983), and making tonal discrimations (Kimura 1967). These processing specialisations can account for the non-verbal and prosodic abnormalities that may follow RH lesion in a simple and direct way. The remaining deficits, however, need careful evaluation. The evidence of lexical semantic impairment is controversial as many studies investigating lexical impairments have used picture materials and, given the visuospatial disturbances that can follow right hemisphere damage (RHD), the interpretation of errors on such tasks is not unambiguous (Chieffi *et al.* 1989, Varley 1995) .

The presumed lexical deficit of RHD is an example of how an apparently linguistic sign can, in fact, be a consequence of other impairments, i.e. a secondary manifestation, and it is productive to assess whether other components of the RH communicative syndrome may have a similar indirect genesis. Difficulties with non-literal language tasks may not be unique to RHD. Eisenson (1962) in his original description of RHD characteristics, described these patients as having difficulties in completing 'extraordinary' language tasks. Non-literal language tasks, such as joke tests, interpretation of metaphors, and tasks requiring the respondent to go beyond the available literal information to make inferences, are difficult language tasks and place demands on processing systems outside language, for example, the demand for additional attention resources.

Any deficits identified cannot then be unambiguously attributed to specific right hemisphere processing systems: they may simply be due to the effects of more generalised brain damage. The issue of specific or primary language deficit is again important in the consideration of discourse and pragmatic deficits. Discourse deficits do not occur uniquely in RHD. MacDonald (1993) has pointed out the similarities in discourse behaviour of closed head injury and RHD patients. Discourse deficits also occur in other disorders where cognitive abnormalities are seen as the underlying cause (e.g. schizophrenia, high-level autism and Williams syndrome). Discourse and conversation represent the highest level of demand on communicative systems, requiring not only linguistic encoding, but cohesion across sentences, management of topic, and making contributions appropriate to the listener and the situation. They also require planning of communicative goals (e.g. the wish to signal that one is friendly, seek to inform, to deceive, etc.) and monitoring the success of the plan through listeners' reactions, both verbal and non-verbal. Appropriate communicative behaviour is therefore a complex product of many cognitive systems, both linguistic and non-linguistic. It is therefore liable to disruption from different sources. Impairment of specific discourse structuring and conversational interactional rules (see Hampshire and Mogford-Bevan, this volume, Chapter 4.2) would represent primary pragmatic disability, but secondary, 'knock-on' pragmatic disabilities would result from disruptions to linguistic systems of grammar and lexis, and also impairment of non-language cognitive systems such as those involved in developing plans and monitoring their implementation (McTear 1985a).

The case study reported below revolves around the issue of whether the patient had a specific language (discourse/conversational) disorder, or whether his communicative difficulties stemmed from the non-language cognitive sequelae of his brain lesion. The issue is not only of theoretical importance but also of clinical relevance. Intervention which is directed at the source of a disorder is more likely to be effective than intervention which is directed at the secondary consequences of the disorder. In the case of RHD, if the discourse abnormalities stem from underlying cognitive impairments rather than any particular difficulty in structuring language above the level of the sentence, then intervention would be better targeted at the cognitive impairments, rather than at the behaviours which are consequent upon them.

Subject information

RM is a retired senior manager in an insurance company. He lives with his wife and is involved in local church, sporting and social activities. At the time of this investigation he was 68 years old. Two years prior to the assessments and interventions reported here, he suffered a right hemispheric lesion. A CT scan revealed a large right haemorrhagic lesion, which involved cortical white matter, but spared much of the cortex. There was also a possible old left hemispheric lesion close to the anterior pole of the left lateral ventricle. RM's medical history, and also the history given by RM and his wife, gave no report of any previous neurological illness, but it may well be that RM did have bilateral brain lesions and although he showed evidence of discourse and conversational abnormalities, he may not be typical of the RHD population in all respects. RM was premorbidly unambiguously right-handed.

Following his cerebrovascular accident (CVA), RM presented with a range of difficulties including a left hemiparesis, left hemianaesthesia, left hemianopia, a range of impairments linked to disturbed visuo-spatial processing (constructional apraxia, dressing apraxia, neglect dyslexia), neglect, and anosagnosia (for example, he rated himself as 60% effective as a communicator prior to his CVA, and 80% effective post-CVA). In addition, he was reported to have concentration problems and discourse and conversational abnormalities. Prior to any intervention or informational counselling (i.e. counselling which provides the client and family with information on the possible consequences of a RH lesion and feedback on assessment results), RM's spouse was asked to complete a questionnaire regarding changes in communicative performance. This questionnaire was administered because, whereas it is usually straightforward to discriminate aphasic impairments from normal language, the dividing line between conversational disability and the range of normal conversational performance is less clear. RM's spouse was able to give an exceptionally clear characterisation of RH communicative disorder. She wrote:

> Talks more, and talks faster. Wants to tell often irrelevant details. Sometimes starts in the middle of a story and expects the listener to know what went before. Moves off at a tangent in a conversation if a sudden thought diverts his attention.

RM was seen for 10 sessions of therapy prior to his discharge from hospital. Sessions focused on informational counselling, administration of the Right Hemisphere Language Battery (Bryan 1994), and intervention directed at reducing the length of his talk turns in conversation and monitoring his listener for signs of discomfort. Evaluation of the effectiveness of this intervention was not possible as RM was discharged soon after the programme's onset. RM received no speech and language therapy over the following 22 months.

Two years post-onset, RM began to attend a university clinic once a week. At this point, RM had maintained many of his pre-morbid social and church activities with his wife's support. His visuospatial, neglect, and anosognosic difficulties had not resolved over the intervening months. With regard to communication, although quantitative analyses were not possible, RM's difficulties with eye contact and excessively lengthy talk turns had resolved to some degree. The Right Hemisphere Language Battery was re-administered, and his score had remained stable over the intervening 2 years. RM's scores (converted to standardised scores) on the various sub-tests, together with the mean scores of Bryan's non-brain damaged (NBD) controls and RHD group are presented in Table 4.3.1.

Table 4.3.1 RM's scores on the Right Hemisphere Language Battery

Test	RM	Control (Bryan)	RHD (Bryan)
Metaphor picture	49/70	61/70	45/70
Metaphor written	52/70	59/70	45/70
Comprehension of inference	43/70	48/70	43/70
Appreciation of humour	57/70	63/70	45/70
Lexical semantic test	62/70	62/70	44/70
Production of emphatic stress	50/70	57/70	43/70
Discourse analysis	63/70	68/70	43/70

Inspection of the scores reveals that apart from scores on the Metaphor Picture Test and the Comprehension of Inferred Meaning, RM's scores lie nearer to those of the control group than Bryan's RHD group. Whereas all the mean scores of Bryan's RHD group lie between 0 and –1 standard deviation, only the two above-mentioned of RM's scores fall in this range. Of particular note are RM's scores on the Discourse Analysis rating scale. Despite his wife's clear report of disordered discourse (and also the data presented below), RM's test score was close to normal. However, it is important to note that the title of this sub-test is misleading. Rather than 'discourse analysis' (a title which implies a full analysis of data, as in Stubbs 1983), it is a checklist assessment in which patient behaviours are scored along a number of pre-selected dimensions. Because full linguistic analyses demand both time and considerable skill from clinicians, the inclusion of a checklist is fully justified from a clinical perspective. The difficulty with such rating scales, however, is that the pre-selected dimensions do not always match the patient's areas of impairment.

RM therefore does not appear to perform in ways typical of RHD patients. One might argue that his possible bilateral damage may be an important factor here, but the fact that he performs at a level superior to unilaterally damaged RH patients makes this unlikely. It may be the unusual nature of his RH brain pathology, with cortical sparing, that is the relevant factor. Whatever the source of the difference, it becomes clear that variability and lack of homogeneity of 'syndrome' characteristics is as an important factor in acquired discourse abnormalities as it is in aphasia (Caramazza 1985).

Investigations: preliminary observations

The first element in intervention was to characterise the nature of RM's conversational and discourse disability. RM had no motor speech or phonological encoding problems. He had occasional lexical retrieval difficulties, but these were not remarkable given his age and the presence of brain pathology. On a test which required the subject to produce an opposite to a stimulus word (Varley 1991), RM scored at a level equivalent to NBD controls (RM 31/36, NBD mean 31.3). Grammatical structure was often hypercomplex, with embedding and complex verb phrase structures in evidence. In terms of language comprehension, RM responded appropriately in conversation, although he had difficulties retaining new information or instructions, particularly if they were unsupported by context. On a test of lexical–semantic comprehension which required the subject to select an opposite to a stimulus word (Varley 1991), RM again performed at a level equivalent to controls (RM 35/36, NBD mean 35.1). Formal language assessments were limited by RM's visual perceptual problems. The reliance of many tests on pictorial materials would introduce a significant non-language confound in RM's case.

Examples of RM's discourse are given in Transcript 1 (Table 4.3.2). The first is from spontaneous conversation, and the second from a more constrained task, where RM is asked to describe an elephant. In the first extract, the length of RM's turn is noticeable (and, in fact, the turn went on for longer than the extract shows). Throughout this turn, RM made no eye contact with his listener. Also noteworthy are the processing demands placed on the listener in order to understand RM. The listener has previously asked a question regarding RM's stroke, and has certain expectations of the likely content of RM's response to such a question. 'Scripts and schemas' (Rumelhart 1980) allow previous experience and stored knowledge to be used to predict what is likely to happen in a situation or in a particular talk exchange. They permit reduction in information processing as, to some extent, the receiver of information can scan information to check for congruence with schema and script expectations. Where script expectations are not met, processing demands on the listener (e.g. demand for attentional resources) are increased. RM begins with a topic which is to a degree congruent with the question asked. But there is then a gradual topic drift, leading to a very marked unsignalled topic shift (carol singing). This is then followed by the phrase '*have to be aware of*' which was frequent in RM's discourse, together with other stereotypes of form. RM may use stereotypes as floor-holders while he tries to regain his direction in conversation. Following the stereotype, there is another marked topic shift, but this time into a piece of narrative, perhaps a story that is frequently told by RM. The presence of the video camera during the recording of this sample may also have influenced the topic change. RM shows an association of ideas, which is not inhibited, from being videotaped now, to being videotaped on a previous occasion (the Birmingham conference). In addition to stereotypes of form, RM also had stereotypes of topic. Whereas the stereotypes of form were not conscious strategies, some of the stereotypes of topic most certainly were. One notable example was of RM initiating interaction with the therapist on three consecutive weeks with the opener '*What do you think of the interact* (= Internet)?'. The availability of this strategy to consciousness was revealed in questioning RM, who reported that he was not at all interested in the Internet, but had worked out that this was a contemporary and technical topic which would show his interlocutor that he was in touch with current affairs and able to deal with abstract ideas. A similar account of stereotypes of form is suggested by Perkins *et al.* (1995) in an analysis of the discourse of a patient with a closed head injury. The authors suggest that their patient's stereotypes represent an attempt at a repair strategy to remedy threatened derailing of the conversation.

Table 4.3.2 Transcript 1 (^ = pause)

Sample 1: conversation
   Therapist: *What difficulties has the stroke left you with?*

RM: *^ ^ The difficulties seems to be ^ to come to a realisation that that this has happened | that I've got to overcome this left foot ^ handicap | and now I'm sure thanks to the ebr work you've done that I'm now beginning to read properly | I couldn't read the newspaper | as you know | um and I got very concerned in ways that I couldn't see the news | I couldn't read my daily paper | which was (1 syllable) most part of my life | I was | I didn't see other things | I don't think I missed out on other things | I think that's | I don't know how much more Margaret has had to do for me | because I've just been in the world of people helping me | teaching me | and prepared to go to some trouble if I will concentrate | and accept | but I think its taught me to keep my humour | and | and believe in God | which I (Inaudible) every day | and look at other people I see | because sometimes I used to think that people | that things happened to people because of their own care-lessness and this sort of ^ smoke and drinking and what-have-you and stupidity | and | one of our friends down the road has had a bad stroke | and his mouth running away | and we went to the clinic the other night | and and there he was in a pretty bad way | and it's taught me that ebr there are some (2 syllables) people who need help | and when I started in the carols | singing | all choir people were singing | and suddenly I was singing Silent Night | and I thought I'm singing | and then I thought of course I'm singing | so it's made me realise that people do have these things happen to them | and it's not their fault | Its something that ebr you've got to be ebr aware of | you've got to try to be more tolerant | and you've got to try hard to accept what other things are happening to people isn't their fault | more than the stupid things like smoking and drinking | and those kind of things | which I consider rather stupid | I suppose that similarly I should not have worked so hard | ^ mentally | and perhaps I haven't got the ability to do things | and now regional manager is coming on Tuesday night next week | and I remember now about oh | ^ I don't know for time | but about 3 years before I retired | we went to a conference in a hotel | and the ebr it was very intense | the video | not the video | this kind of work we'd done | and we all had to do certain tests | and it was all for the company quite advanced | and it was very ultra-modern | and Birmingham manager | he had to go home | he was younger than me by about 6 years | and I helped pack his clothes | and he said that he just couldn't absorb it all | I then spent that evening trying to do a project | and it finished up by more-or-less morning time asking the regional manager to make sure that I'd done it reasonably well | because he was responsible for the whole conference | and I didn't want to let him down | and he spent half an hour an hour going over it with me | and I'd always considered myself equal to him |*

Sample 2: word definition
an elephant is an animal | one of the biggest animals in the ebr world of | um | animal world | it can be ebr ^ very ebr ^ cross | can be troublesome if it's not guided carefully | if it's not used properly | so that the ebr purpose of the elephant has got to be respected and can't just be ebr | looked upon

Table 4.3.2 (contd)

---

as something that is useful | *and when you compare this to the ehr* | ^
other | ^ *actions the elephant does like pull large trees or even heavy*
weights | *ehr they can be extremely helpful useful creatures* | ^ *but you*
must remember as an elephant they are limited to ability that they are
given as a task | *that's the elephant* |

Phase 1: Language-oriented investigation and therapy

The initial phase of intervention examined two possible hypotheses regarding the source of the underlying impairment. The first of these was a hypothesis regarding the processing styles of the left and right hemisphere (Levy 1974), and the second, a theory which has been influential in the study of autism, that of theory of mind (Baron-Cohen *et al.* 1985). The hypothesis of different processing styles of the two hemispheres suggests that the left hemisphere is a specialised analytic and sequential processor, particularly suited to the processing of phonology and grammar because of its expertise in combining small units into larger ones and then computing their value. The right hemisphere is seen as a holistic or gestalt processor, hence its specialisation in the processing of complex visuospatial forms. The language manifestations of RHD have been interpreted in the light of this dichotomy. RHD patients failed in language tasks where integration of information into a coherent whole was required; in discourse they failed because of difficulties in making individual sentences coalesce into coherent discourse and their contributions appropriate to the total context of the listener and the topic. They failed in non-literal language tasks such as inference, because of failure to go beyond the linguistic information and integrate this with other stored knowledge about the world.

The investigation of the hypothesis of a failure of integrative processing underlying RM's communicative difficulties used materials developed by Sharkey and Sharkey (1990), in a study which investigated reading development in normal children. Subjects were presented with a paragraph which ended with a non-word, and were required to select the meaning of the non-word from a choice of four items. Selection of the correct item required integration of the local information of the final sentence with the global information of the rest of the passage. Distractor items were an unrelated word, a response which was globally but not locally correct, and finally one which was locally correct but did not integrate with the information in the main passage (see Figure 4.3.1). Passages were in full view and also read aloud to RM. He scored 15/20 on the task, with all his errors being global ones, i.e. he attended to the total context, but not the local information. This result is discouraging to the gestalt hypothesis. The score may represent a failure of integration of all information, but RM was aware of the global information but not the particular.

The pupils filed into the classroom and sat down. They got out their books and pens. The teacher asked the children to be quiet. He was going to set them some exercises. He picked up the **gennish**.

(a) phone   (b) blackboard   (c) chalk   (d) net

Figure 4.3.1 Sharkey and Sharkey (1990): example test item.

The second hypothesis to be examined was that his difficulties may have reflected a disorder of theory of mind. This hypothesis has been influential in investigations of autism and suggests that the communication impairments, impaired social relationships and ritualistic behaviour of individuals with autism may be due to a failure to attribute mental states to others, or to understand the contents of another individual's mind. Possession of a theory of mind is essential for communication (and for social cognition). Knowledge that others' minds do not contain the same information as your own sets up the need for communication, and the moment-to-moment planning of discourse requires evaluation of what the listener currently knows. Shields *et al.* (1996) have shown that children with autism, and also children with semantic–pragmatic language difficulties, show performances on a neuropsychological test battery which are consistent with a pattern of right hemispheric dysfunction. **Theory of mind** tasks (Happe 1991, Wimmer and Perner 1983) were slightly adapted to make them more appropriate to an adult subject and then administered to RM to assess whether an acquired lesion to the right hemisphere also resulted in failures on theory of mind tasks. The tasks used were first-order false belief and deception tests, and second-order false belief and deception tests. An example of a first-order false belief is an adapted version of the Smarties test. The patient and the tester looked at a pill bottle, which, instead of containing tablets, held buttons. The patient was asked 'if somebody else came into the room, what would they think is in the bottle?' The correct response requires the subject to realise that another's mental state is different from their own. In addition to the test question, the subject is asked a control or reality question ('what is really in the bottle?') to demonstrate their answer to the first question show awareness of a false belief, rather than perhaps a simple forgetting of what actually is in the bottle. RM performed well on these tasks, even to the level of a complex second-order deception task (see Figure 4.3.2).

RM's performance on the theory of mind tasks suggested that he was able to judge what someone else might be thinking, although the moment-to-moment calculation of listeners' knowledge is not tapped by these static tasks. It was felt that neither the theory of mind hypothesis nor the gestalt processing one provided an adequate theoretical basis to design an intervention programme for RM.

Bill has just robbed a bank and he is making his getaway. The police are after him. He meets his brother Bob. He says to Bob 'Don't let the police find me'. He runs and hides in the church. The police arrive. They've looked everywhere for Bill except the park and the church. They ask Bob 'Where is Bill? Is he in the park or the church?' The police recognise Bob and know that he is Bill's brother and will try to save him. They expect him to lie and wherever he tells them to look, they will look in the other place. But Bob is very clever and wants to save his brother. He knows that the police do not trust him.

Where will Bob tell them to look?	*church*
Why does he tell them that?	*because they wouldn't believe.*
	Whatever he says they'll not believe,
	so if he says he'll be there, they'll
	believe the opposite
Where will the police look if he says that?	*park*
Where is Bill hiding really?	*church*

Figure 4.3.2 Second-order deception theory of mind task (Happe 1991, Wimmer and Perner 1983), with RM's responses.

The only obvious route in intervention at this point was to revert to a therapeutic programme based on attacking RM's behavioural deficits. Three behavioural objectives were identified:

- monitoring redundancy and irrelevance in others' and his own discourse
- inhibiting his own confabulatory and verbose output
- awareness of the structuring of discourse through work on narratives and metalinguistic awareness of the content and order of key propositions (Kintsch and van Dijk 1978).

The monitoring programme moved through stages of off-line evaluation and editing of written paragraphs generated by the therapist for inappropriacies, to transcripts of his own narratives. The evaluation and editing process was then applied to on-line judgements of first the clinician's spoken discourse for irrelevancies and then finally to on-line evaluation of his own discourse.

Once successful on-line monitoring of self was established, the programme moved on to first inhibiting his output once he had gone off track. Despite RM's ability to monitor his own discourse failure (he would often signal non-verbally to the therapist that he knew he was talking 'junk'), he had great difficulty moving from recognition into action to repair the breakdown. Ways of initiating a repair were suggested and modelled to RM (e.g. *I've lost my thread. Where was I?*'). The second objective therefore aimed to develop inhibition of confabulatory output in real-time speaking. As he seemed to having difficulty generating an internal action plan, an external prompt of a television remote control was used to remind RM to switch off his output when he recognised inappropriacies.

The third element in this phase of intervention was to develop RM's awareness of the internal structure of discourse. Simple narrative stories were used. A loose story grammar approach (Mandler and Johnson 1977) was used to develop metalinguistic awareness of the structure of the narrative. For example, the 'dog story' (Lees 1993, and see Figure 4.3.3) was divided into two main episodes (obtaining the meat and losing the meat), each of which was sub-divided into a setting, an initiating event, and a response. The second episode also included a consequence and a coda (Roth and Spekman 1986). RM and the therapist linked the story structure with propositions within the story and then RM practised the retelling of the story with various prompts to the story structure in view.

A dog is walking along past a butcher's shop. In a dustbin, he finds a piece of meat and he grabs this and runs off home with it. In order to get home, he has to cross a bridge over a canal. As he walks over the bridge, he sees his reflection in the water below and thinks that it is another dog who appears to have an enormous piece of meat in his mouth, much bigger than his own. And so he snaps at the reflection, and in so doing, drops his own piece of meat into the water. He goes home hungry.

Episode 1 (obtaining the meat)
Setting   *dog walk*
Initiating event   *finds meat*
Response   *steals meat*

Episode 2 (losing the meat)
Setting   *dog cross canal*
Initiating event   *sees reflection*
Response   *snaps at reflection*
Consequence   *loses meat*
Coda   *hungry*

Figure 4.3.3 The dog story.

Results

The first stage of intervention was considered effective. RM became adept at monitoring his own discourse in on-line situations. The difficulty in getting him to move from identification of failure to the initiation of a repair remained difficult. The external prompts did remind RM to inhibit his output. This is illustrated in using an ideational fluency task (e.g. how many uses can you think of for a brick), before intervention and during intervention with the external prompt (Table 4.3.3). The external prompt therefore results in some improvements. Performance following intervention appears better. Primarily it takes 23 words to describe a single function of a brick versus 116 also to describe a single function of a brick. The first sample also contains some characteristic errors: repeated use of sentence form ('without it collapsing/being soft/being useless'), and the intrusion of a irrelevant idea ('if you get these words correct'). But a very serious issue begins to emerge with the changes in the discourse output. The purpose of an ideational fluency task is to see how many different ideas an individual can generate. Intervention directed at language has no effect on the generativity of RM's ideas. In pre- and post-intervention measures he can realise only one (obvious) use for a brick. Removal of RM's linguistic, confabulatory 'camouflage' results in exposure of a stark underlying deficit in idea generation. At this point there was an issue of the acceptability of the new (and supposedly improved) discourse for RM and his wife. Both expressed a preference for the confabulatory discourse which obscured the cognitive deficits.

Table 4.3.3 Ideational fluency task (uses for a brick)

Pre-intervention

a ^ | a brick is a solid piece of material | that is ebr often used for ^ providing some kind of object | that is ebr useful | and can be ebr ^ um ^ | used mostly in the building trade | and that it provides material that is solid and firm and ebr | has many many ways of ^ | providing ^ this material um without it collapsing | without it being soft | without it being useless | um that ebr brick is ebr usually mostly used on the building sites | where the person has to achieve a certain amount of ebr uses | certain amount of ^ uses for the building trade | and if you ebr | if you get these words correct you can then build up um ^ | the way in which the material is going to be of ^ ebr purpose |

During intervention

I can think of a use of a housebrick | is for making a wall ^ | or ^ making a building ^ | or making it ^ worthwhile purpose |

The results of intervention directed at story structure showed a change in performance after intervention. This is illustrated by before and after examples of RM's retelling of the dog story (Table 4.3.4). On a number of measures there appear to be improvements following intervention. The post-intervention attempt is shorter (78 words versus 112), contains more propositions core to the story (4 versus 3), and fewer extraneous propositions (0 versus 5, this latter measure and subsequent measures exclude the final section of the transcript from 'I was just gonna say', which has nothing to do with the retelling of the dog story). There are a number of other linguistic characteristics of the first sample which reflect the greater amount of empty, confabulating language contained within it. It is syntactically more complex (78% of main clauses contain embedded clauses in the pre-intervention sample, compared with 50% in the second) and contains a greater number of items whose reference is not specific (36% of phrase heads are deictic in the first sample versus 19% in the second). Non-specific reference and embedding are useful design characteristics for confabulating language. Non-specific reference permits the utterance to be 'multipurpose' as the content is not tightly constrained. Embedding can result in output, so fulfilling the social obligation to respond to an interlocutor's utterance, without commitment to many specific propositions (e.g. 'I think that, when you consider the situation, and I have often felt this in the past that ... '). Such superficially complex language may also provide the speaker with time to formulate a plan of what to say next.

Table 4.3.4 The dog story, before and after intervention

Pre-intervention

the animal um was ehr coming along ^ the road | where-ever | and he saw this um piece of ehr meat that he felt would be very acceptable | and um made ehr ehr grab to absorb this | um and run off with it | but of course | ehr he didn't ehr remember that ehr you have got to be ehr more skilful | you've got to be aware of ehr how must ehr get yourself in the right position | how you must hold your mouth to ehr to get the ehr ^ part that you are requiring | and having done that | you've also got to be sure that you are able to um use the facility | um rather than just hopefully um expect that it is going to be there if you happen to be fortunate | I think that ^ | I was just gonna say that the only thing that I can add to that is that um | in effect I've got to think out as you try showed me before that | or am I getting a bit further along now | where I'm talking about other people | I must try to remember the need for conversation is is two | now the word you gave me is twofold | that it's not just got to be one-way | that it's the | oh dear | I knew the word and I've gone and lost it |
(Notice the appearance of the '*to be aware of*' stereotype at the point where the retelling of the story has gone off track)

Post-intervention

This dog to get home had to cross a river | and crossing the river | he saw a reflection in the river | the juicy piece of meat | and he was hungry | so he opened his mouth to grab the piece of meat that he could see in the reflection in the river and | instead of grabbing the meat | he lost the meat in the river | so he finished up with no meat | that's a concise story of the dog |

Despite the apparent improvement, the post-intervention attempt remains, despite multiple attempts and training on this one story, a poor attempt at retelling of the dog story because much of the first episode, that the dog already has a piece of meat in his mouth, is omitted. Gains were also very fragile. Attempts to improve the internal structure of narratives failed to produce transfer to new and untrained stories.

Phase 2: Cognitively-oriented investigation and therapy

In the second phase of assessment, the hypothesis driving intervention was that RM's communicative difficulties resulted from a relatively intact linguistic system 'camouflaging' underlying cognitive abnormalities. Hence the communicative signs represented secondary difficulties; RM's underlying impairment lay in the cognitive systems which underpinned the use of language in ongoing interactions. This hypothesis was influenced by the suggestion of MacDonald (1993) that RHD patients are similar in their communicative signs to patients with closed head injury, many of whom suffer from lesions to the frontal lobes and have impairments of executive functions. Executive functions are the planning and monitoring functions that supervise other cognitive modules such as language and working memory (Shallice 1988). Knowledge of executive functions is still at an early stage, and there is little to guide the clinician seeking principled intervention of impairments in this area. Norman and Shallice (1980) address some elements of executive functioning, in particular in their model of the supervisory attentional system (SAS). They suggest that behaviour can be governed by schemata or stored knowledge and an associated 'contention scheduling device' which resolves conflicts between different schemata. At a higher level, the SAS monitors the success of behaviour and, where schema-driven behaviour is resulting in failure, or where the situation is novel and no pre-stored schema exists, it intervenes and organises new adaptive behaviours. Making a speculative link to RM's communicative behaviour, he may perform well where a pre-existing schema is available and appropriate to a situation (e.g. greeting routines, retelling a well-known story), but in novel situations where schemata are not available, RM falls back on confabulating and stereotyped language which masks the underlying difficulties. An important characteristic of discourse abnormalities such as RM's is that they are subject to a large degree of context-conditioned variability. Whereas an aphasic individual's difficulties with grammar and lexicon are likely to be relatively consistent across contexts, RM's behaviour will appear normal in situations which are governed by established scripts and schemas, but impairments will emerge where novel behaviour is demanded.

This hypothesis was tested by administering to RM a set of tasks which were diverse, but linked by a common thread of requiring processing of novel information or resisting a habitual way of responding. None of the tasks are 'pure' tests of novelty. The nature of **executive** functions is that they sit on top of other processing systems. All the tasks involve variable degrees of language processing. Non-linguistic novelty tasks, e.g. Guilford's circles test (Guilford 1967), were avoided because of RM's visual difficulties. These tasks and their results are summarised below.

Auditory stroop

A **Stroop task** is one in which there is a conflict between perceptual and linguistic information (Stroop 1935). The usual stroop procedure involves responding to colour words whose ink colour is incompatible with the colour name (e.g. *blue* written in red ink). Because of RM's visual difficulties, an auditory analogue of colour stroop was used (Green and Barber 1981). Stroop stimuli were the words *man* and *woman* spoken by male and female speakers. In the stroop by perceptual criterion, RM was required to respond to speaker gender, and in the semantic criterion task, he was required to respond to the word. Perceptual criterion tasks are generally more difficult because they require suppression of the habitual response, i.e. responding to the semantic information of a word. There were also two control tasks both using the neutral words *dog/table*: on the first a male speaker was heard and the subject was required to respond to one of the words; the second was a voice identification task, where a male and a female speaker produced the neutral words and the subject was required to respond to the male/female speaker irrespective of what was said. The control tasks excluded voice identification difficulties as a possible confound of RHD results, and also acted as training trials where responding by both perceptual and semantic criterion was established.

RM was matched with a NBD control. The control subject performed the tests once. The control subject made no errors on control tasks and the stroop by semantic criterion. On the stroop by perceptual criterion, the control subject performed at 90% accuracy. RM was given the tests across a number of sessions. Only data from trials where RM was able to report the response criterion at the end of the trial were analysed so as to eliminate the effect of simple forgetting of the task instruction from the results. RM made no errors on the first control test. Accuracy scores for the remaining tests were voice gender identification 90% accuracy, stroop by semantic criterion 94% accuracy, stroop by perceptual criterion 77% accuracy. These results suggest that RM had particular difficulties on the perceptual stroop task where he was unable to suppress the habitual response to semantic information.

Novel and dead metaphors

Difficulty in interpreting metaphors has been identified as an element in the RHD symptomatology. RM's results on the Right Hemisphere Language Battery indicated some difficulties with the Picture Metaphor Test, although this result may be confounded by RM's visuoperceptual difficulties. The metaphors used in the Right Hemisphere Language Battery are all 'dead' metaphors (e.g. *green fingers*): they are familiar and may well have been learned as compound lexical entries rather than having true non-literal properties. RM was given a set of dead metaphors to interpret and a set of novel ones. He scored 9/10 on dead metaphors and 3/11 on novel metaphors.

Fluency tests

RM was given a series of fluency tests which vary in the degree of novelty of processing demanded. The first task was word fluency via a phonological criterion (words beginning with /f/or/s/). As storage in the phonological output lexicon is believed to be organised via phonological form, this was classified as the least novel task. Word fluency by a semantic criterion (e.g. recall of animal names) requires access to pre-stored information but by a more unusual search criterion. The final fluency test, ideational fluency (e.g. functions of a piece of string) requires the subject to go beyond stored information and to generate new ideas. RM's scores on the fluency tests were: phonological criterion 29 (control 30, Hodges 1994), semantic criterion 31 (control 54, Varley 1995), ideational 1. The pattern of results indicates a gradual falling off of performance from normal (where norms are available) as the novelty of the task increases.

Hypothetical questions

A series of hypothetical questions was devised (e.g. 'what would happen if we did not record or celebrate birthdays?'). These questions, like ideational fluency tasks, require novel reasoning. As might be predicted from the ideational fluency score, RM found the task difficult and they had to be abandoned. Instead of addressing the question, RM's responses represented questioning of the premises of the task (e.g. 'I don't think you are the type of person who would forget birthdays').

RM's performance across these tasks suggested that he had difficulty moving away from habitual processing to processing of novel information. The tasks varied greatly in terms of their language-loading – with relatively little beyond lexical processing required on stroop and word fluency, but discourse comprehension and production on some others. Despite the differential language-loading, the novelty effect appeared across tasks. The data from these assessments provided some support that intervention directed at the complex area of executive functions might be worthwhile. These functions are not unitary and, as a first stage in intervention, the process of sustained attention was identified as a target for intervention. It is not suggested that RM's difficulties lay solely in the area of attention, but it was believed that sustained attention was a prerequisite for other abilities such as planning and problem solving. The decision to target attention was supported by comments from RM and his spouse that he often became distracted by associated ideas or by irrelevant external stimuli.

A modified version of a successful attention training programme reported by Robertson *et al.* (1995) was planned. This is a simple programme which moves through the stages of giving the subject feedback on performance on a particular task and pointing out failures. Then, in the metacognitive stage, the therapist explains the importance of sustained attention for performance and the therapeutic strategy is explained. The strategy involves moving from therapist-generated attention alerters ('attend'), to fading of the therapist and initiation by the patient of self-alerters. First these are external, but are then faded, so that an internal self-alert strategy is established. In the planned intervention with RM, the therapy would follow the procedure given by Robertson *et al.*, with the practice tasks emphasising narrative discourse. Sadly, while the baseline measures for this intervention were being taken, RM had a further CVA, rendering this approach to therapy inappropriate

Summary and conclusions

This case study reports the case of RM, who suffered a large right hemisphere lesion, with possible bilateral involvement. His lesion left him with difficulties in discourse and conversation. It is argued that these difficulties do not represent a primary discourse deficit, but stem from cognitive deficits that followed from his lesion. A theme of this case study has been that successful intervention requires an adequate conceptualisation of the source of deficits. Intervention directed at secondary manifestations of his problem led to superficial and transient changes in behaviour. RM's difficulties are manifest in contexts which are not routine, where his difficulties in the assembly of new behaviours become apparent.

Acknowledgements

I would like to thank Amanda Carr and Kate Sisum for help in data collection, and Dariel Merrills for assistance with the metaphor task. Special thanks go to RM and his wife for their enthusiastic support and involvement throughout the many phases of this project.

Chapter 4.4
Afterword

JAMES LAW

By definition the aetiologies of the two cases RM and N are different. We have a strong suggestion that many of RM's difficulties are caused by his right hemisphere lesion in the first instance, even though his assessed language does not appear to reflect this. N, in contrast, presents as a relatively characteristic language-delayed child with some associated autistic behaviours. His language difficulties seem to have resolved spontaneously and the difficulties he experiences in interaction are all that remain of his earlier impairment. Not surprisingly, given the way that these studies were set up independently of each other, we have rather inconsistent levels of information. It would have been interesting, for example, to have access to the results from a range of tasks designed to access skills associated with the right or the left hemisphere for both cases to see the extent to which the right hemisphere is implicated. It would also have been interesting to report the individuals' responses to the same range of language measures and to the same theory of mind tasks.

It appears that Hampshire and Mogford-Bevan's subject had an intact perception of others and given this it would be reasonable to assume that the problems experienced by the child are more discrete and therefore less intractable than those experienced by Varley's subject. But we are still left with the question of how a child from a family background with 'optimal' input could have this level of difficulty in the first place and particularly how such a difficulty could occur in isolation. In fact the evidence for the discrete nature of this difficulty is somewhat equivocal given that he had a history of language delay, a relatively low score on the Test for Reception of Grammar and a history of poorly developed symbolic skills. It is commonly observed that such children learn to perform much more efficiently on highly structured assessments such as the TROG relative to their performance in context where the options may not be so circumscribed.

Even so, we are then faced with the problem of explaining how such

235

a marked problem as it appears can be improved over such a comparatively short period of time. It may, of course, be that the overall level of
input which he had received in the unit may have provided him with the
necessary sub-skills such as listening and understanding which are then
triggered by the right intervention at the right time. Is it possible then
to speak of a pragmatic 'readiness', and how can we define this quality
so that it could be recognised and exploited by others?

It could, of course, be that a child with such a specific pragmatic
profile may be a great rarity. The 'semantic pragmatic' profile to which
clinical reference is more commonly made may be the norm and
certainly from clinical experience these children are often seen as
having pervasive problems which respond in only a limited fashion to
therapy. Many would refer to such children as being on the autistic spec-
trum. As discussed in Chapter 4.1, the fact that it may be possible to
isolate children with discrete pragmatic difficulties is interesting for
what it tells us about the possible dissociation between pragmatic and
other language skills.

Varley's case presents with a much more obvious pattern of structural
language problems in association with the pragmatic aspects of the
breakdown. Indeed, her conclusion post-therapy is that her client had a
much more pervasive central deficit. This is convincing, but we are still
left wondering whether arguments regarding pragmatic deficits following right brain damage go any way to explaining the presenting symptoms given his performance on the assessment designed to pick up just
these phenomena.

There are a number of comparisons to be made in the therapy itself.
From what we have seen, Hampshire and Mogford-Bevan adopted a
behavioural approach to introduce the polar interrogative and then
moved to a phase of social skills training (**metapragmatics**) with a view
to the child generalising out into the context in the classroom. By
contrast, Varley starts with a social skills approach and then becomes
more specific. Although Varley notes improvements, it is clear that
Hampshire and Mogford-Bevan's case improves to a far greater extent.
It may be that we simply do not have enough information to compare
the cases effectively. If RM had much more pervasive problems, of which
the problems in handling discourse were only one manifestation, these
results are hardly surprising.

What connections can then be made with regard to therapy for adults
and children with this type of disorder? The first concerns the general
context in which the individual exists. Pragmatic skills cannot by their
nature be taught out of context. Although the therapy time for
Hampshire and Mogford-Bevan's case was relatively short, the learning
environment of the school and the expectations placed upon the child
in a such a context provide more opportunities for extension and generalisation than would therapy sessions alone. RM is provided with very

specific tasks associated with monitoring discourse in textual form but it is not clear whether others were involved in carrying out this type of activity with him. Interestingly the result of therapy is a reduction in irrelevant output. Varley then became aware that this was serving to 'camouflage' a deficit in idea generation, suggesting that RM's pragmatic deficit may in fact be a strategy adopted to mask difficulties in other areas. So while both therapies reduce extraneous utterances they lead to different conclusions being drawn about the client.

Another important issue is that of assessment. Although, as Hampshire and Mogford-Bevan indicate, traditional assessment techniques do not help pinpoint the nature of the impairment they remain important in that they can contribute to the differential diagnosis. To get at the nature of the problem it is clearly important to examine the individual's capacity to interact effectively with a range of other speakers and preferably in different contexts. It may be that these factors play a large part in determining whether someone has a conversational difficulty. In the case of both the adult and the child it may be as appropriate to look at what could be considered as an appropriate interactive strategy on the part of the hearer as much as the speaker. Hampshire and Mogford-Bevan's use of conversational analysis, a system of classifying discourse without using any predetermined criteria, offers a promising technique for getting at the surface manifestations of the child's disability and one which is finding favour in both developmental and acquired fields. It is questionable whether it would have revealed more than was found with the 'dog story' in the case of RM, because the extent of the intended communication once it was stripped of the surface manifestations was so limited.

An area of central importance to communication as a whole is that of the motivation of the client. It was clear that Hampshire and Mogford-Bevan managed to engage N and encourage him to modify his behaviour. This would be considered a normal part of the therapeutic process and there is nothing in N's behaviour which would suggest that he did not accept this. By contrast we start off with RM's anosognosia: he believed that his communication skills had improved after his stroke, directly contrary to the judgement of his spouse. It would be reasonable to assume that this would make motivation for change a major issue. The perceived purpose of therapy is an integral part of the therapeutic process, an obstacle which may be inherently easier to overcome when working with children who spend a large part of their lives in a learning environment, one in which they are frequently being asked to use their language to reflect on what they have learned and on how it is communicated. It seems likely that metapragmatic skills are a prerequisite for therapy in both adult and child domains and it is just these skills which are likely to be affected in pragmatic disorders.

Where the connections become weaker is in our understanding of what it means to have a conversational or pragmatic impairment in child or adulthood. There is a danger that we compare the child's behaviour with the adult model, an assumption which is generally acceptable with the adult but much less so for the child. Hampshire and Mogford-Bevan note that adults were much better at compensating for N's difficulties at maintaining conversations. Other children did not have these skills, and this highlights the need to recognise that children's pragmatic skills continue to develop right through school, long after they have acquired the greater part of their grammatical repertoire. The range of acceptability which is broad enough for adults is even wider for children. As our understanding of the development of pragmatic functions increases it may well be that we are able to be more precise about where and when to target therapy.

Part 5:
Postscript

Chapter 5.1
Making new connections: are patterns emerging?

MARIA BLACK

What emerges clearly from a conference such as this is something we have always suspected: the barriers separating those working with children from those working with adults are more historical and institutional than theoretical. As it is argued in the General Introduction to this volume, theoretical shifts have cleared away the more substantial theoretical obstacles. The common ground is considerable and it is worth outlining some of the common strands in how we understand, assess and treat language impairment in both children and adults.

From symptoms to causes

There is fundamental agreement that the best way to understand language impairment is by reference to models of unimpaired processing. These models allow us to move beyond observation and description of symptoms towards explanation in terms of underlying processing representations and mechanisms. The transition is slow and uneven but perceptible.

In spite of the multiplicity and variety of processing models, there are some common assumptions that are consonant with the cases presented here and much of the current literature. First of all, we can think of processing as **modular**, at least in the sense of involving distinct sets of representations and mechanisms with specific properties and patterns of breakdown. It is by reference to these modules that a gross characterisation of impairment is given, as the different sections of this volume show.

However, there is a growing consensus that processing and impairment cannot be characterised only in terms of individual modules. Language processing is a dynamic system where different sources of information and processing mechanisms interact cooperatively in complex ways that are still poorly understood. If we focus only on the individual components of the system we risk losing sight of some of its crucial properties as Beer (1996) warns:

> ... if you take a radio set to pieces you can certainly understand how it works, and even build a duplicate that works. But although you may survey all the components, neatly spread out and labelled, you never seem to find the voice. (p. 12)

It is increasingly clear that many impairments in both children and adults precisely involve a breakdown in the information flows or interactions between processing modules, as some of the cases in this volume demonstrate.

For instance, Vance argues that the functioning of one module is a precondition for the establishment of representations in another:

> The auditory processing difficulties have also affected semantic representation. Sometimes when a known word was heard it was not recognised as a word with an existing lexical entry. This prevented the semantic representations from being updated by the additional semantic information gained from hearing words in different contexts. Additionally, there were times when a new word was perceived as being the same as an existing known word. The semantic information relating to the new word become incorporated into the semantic representation of the existing lexical item. (p. 30)

It is not just that phonology is more fundamental because it acts as 'the gateway to language' and phonological processing delivers the input to the other modules. What is crucial is the correlation of different sources of information, which allows 'normal' development to take place. As Hirsh-Pasek *et al.* (1996) say:

> ... the grammar of language is found not just in the syntax ... but in a richly correlated set of cues available in the social context, the prosody, semantics, and morphology ... language comprehension can occur at first only when the cues coming from the semantic, prosodic, syntactic, and social systems are redundantly correlated. In other words, for early comprehension to occur, all the planets, as it were, must be in alignment. (pp. 460–1)

We are still a long way from understanding what 'lack of alignment' means in practice but we might be seeing its consequences in some of the children presented in this volume (see Chapters 3.2 and 4.2). Another instance might be a type of case that was brought up repeatedly in the discussion at the conference: children with phonological problems who produce very few verbs, or predicates in general. Why should phonological problems co-occur with verb problems?

Imagine we do not think of word meanings as pre-established conceptual parcels which are simply associated as individual units with corresponding phonological units. Instead, let's think of word meanings as patterns of activation over conceptual nodes or features, as connectionist models invite us to do (see Rumelhart and McClelland 1986). Some conceptual nodes or features will be 'bundled together' simply by being activated together on a regular basis from a variety of perceptual sources – vision, haptic or kinaesthetic perception. Pre-linguistically, we can perceive a variety of individual objects as such because their parts or features co-occur in space and time on a regular basis. Similarly, perception and motor feedback make us treat some actions that are made up of subparts (e.g. walking, running) as a single action even before we have a single word for each of them. In these cases, there will be a perception-based bundle, 'an item', ready to be put into correspondence with a phonological form.

In other cases perception will just not deliver the right bundles. Without experience with a particular language, we simply would not know which conceptual nodes should be activated at the same time to go with a particular phonological form, especially for many verbs, prepositions, adjectives and functors of different kinds that do not have one-to-one perceptual correlates. The main source of regular coactivation would be coming from the phonological module in that it is the regular connection to a unique phonological form that would primarily tie all the relevant conceptual nodes together. In these cases, being 'an item' in the conceptual system would depend on a regular and functioning connection with the phonological lexicon, and with a functioning phonological processing module. We might speculate that, unless a group of conceptual nodes has enough regular coactivation, it will not function as an item for output purposes. It simply will not be produced as a single word. So if a child has phonological problems that lead to inadequate coactivation of sets of conceptual nodes and there are no other sources of coactivation, then the relevant 'meaning' will not be established either for input or for output purposes.

In the adult case, a regular pattern of coactivation of the relevant conceptual nodes will have been established over the years of language use. What might happen if the flow of activation from the phonological lexicon to the conceptual system is reduced through brain damage? Some patterns of coactivation of conceptual nodes will continue to be reinforced through non-linguistic experience. Others, however, might lose some of the strength of connection due to the lack of coactivation from the phonological system. Eventually, these groups of conceptual nodes will stop being lexical items altogether or not behave reliably as items.

Many phenomena in both 'normal' and impaired language processing have led to the development of more interactive models of lexical access and lexical processing where information flows in parallel rather than serially, and there is **feedback** as well as **feedforward** from one module to another. For instance, it would be hard to explain the phonological similarity that holds between semantic errors and their targets for people with and without aphasia if we did not assume some form of feedback from phonological forms to semantic representations (see Martin *et al*. 1996). In this volume, Best *et al*. (Chapter 2.3) argue that their results may be better understood in terms of connectionist models where

...lexical representations ... consist of distributed patterns of activation across semantic, orthographic and phonological domains. Within these interactive networks, activation of a representation within one domain will tend to evoke the representations within the other. In general, co-activation of parts of representations will tend to strengthen the connections between them. From this perspective, the critical part of our treatment is that it involves simultaneous activation of phonological, semantic and orthographic representations. The more the representations are evoked together the more strongly they will be linked and then this strengthened representation will be more easily evoked. (pp. 127–8)

This more interactive approach applies to all areas of processing: recognition, comprehension, reproduction, production. At each stage in processing, several partially specified representations may be generated in parallel and evaluated with respect to a range of factors (e.g. context plausibility) and assigned different priorities or weeded out entirely (see Tanenhaus 1988, Trueswell *et al.* 1994). All the sources of relevant information are brought to bear on processing even if they are not logically necessary for performance on a particular task.

These insights, which have perhaps been implicit in much clinical practice in the past, are now explicitly incorporated into the assessment and treatment of both children and adults. For instance, the importance of lip-reading information in auditory discrimination is recognised and put to therapeutic use by Vance (Chapter 1.2) and by Morris (Chapter 1.3); orthographic input is used in spoken naming by Best *et al.* (Chapter 2.3); and pictorial input is employed to facilitate and support oral production by Bryan (Chapter 3.2) and by Pethers (Chapter 3.3).

Another theoretical assumption that is becoming common in work with children as well as adults is that processing is the product of different types of mechanisms: some are habitual, probabilistic and associative in their nature while others are structure-dependent, combinatorial and symbolic – a distinction Bever (1992) describes as 'the habitual beast' versus 'the structural demon'. Connectionist models are probably better at taming the habitual beasts, while more traditional symbolic and rule-governed models do better with structural demons, though the modelling issue is still hotly debated (see Reilly and Sharkey 1992).

A second distinction, introduced originally by Marslen-Wilson and Tyler (see Tyler 1992), is that between **on-line processes** that are automatic, not under conscious control or available to conscious reflection, and **off-line processes** that underlie our ability to make explicit, more or less conscious, decisions about the properties of linguistic representations.

Although there is still much dispute as to which processes are involved in which task, the distinction is important to clinicians as different processes may well require different forms of assessment and treatment, as it is suggested in the following sections. For instance, Tyler (1992) argues that one of the people with aphasia she studied, RH, has

> no difficulty constructing intermediate representations of an utterance as he hears it. However, when tested on tasks requiring him to make some kind of explicit response to an utterance, either in the form of a sentence–picture match or a judgement, he performs very poorly. (p. 268)

These conceptual tools can be applied to processing in general, irrespective of whether children or adults are involved, and may advance our understanding of what is involved in the performance of particular assessment and therapy tasks.

Identifying the causes

There are striking similarities in the methods of assessment used with both children and adults.

Although the materials and some of the standardised assessements are inevitably different, the **psycholinguistic properties** of the stimuli used in specific tasks are similar. Variables like frequency, imageability, age of acquisition, and operativity are controlled for in studies with both children and adults (see the chapters in Part 2 of this volume).

Similar phonological, semantic, syntactic and morphological properties are taken into account in the selection of stimuli for particular types of tasks. For instance, segmental properties, number and type of syllables, rhyme, and stress patterns are manipulated in a number of studies of auditory processing and lexical retrieval – see for example the chapters by Vance (Chapter 1.2), Morris (Chapter 1.3), Lewis and Speake (Chapter 2.2) and Best *et al.* (Chapter 2.3).

The conceptual properties of single words and the semantic interconnections between words are exploited in testing and therapy with both children and adults (see Chapters 2.2, 2.3, 3.3). Our increasing theoretical understanding of the nature of events and the semantic properties of the predicates that express them has been reflected in testing and the analysis of language produced by children and adults. Factors such as the number of arguments a predicate takes and the thematic roles it assigns have become part of testing and profiling, and more attention has been paid to the systematic relationships between semantic and syntactic structure (see Chapters 3.2 and 3.3 in this volume, and Black *et al.* 1992).

There are similarities in the types of pragmatic properties and types of pragmatic analysis carried out in assessing children and adults. Notions such as relevance, cohesion, initiation, turn-taking and speech acts are applied in both cases (see Chapter 4.2 in this volume, and Lesser and Milroy 1993). Thus, clinicians and researchers working with adults and children employ similar psycholinguistic concepts in selecting stimuli for their tasks and analyse utterances and discourse by reference to similar psycholinguistic parameters. The types of tasks are also similar. Those employed in the studies in this volume could be roughly divided into the following categories in relation to the areas of processing they focus on:

- recognition (auditory and orthographic)
- comprehension
- reproduction
- 'silent' production
- production.

Recognition by children and adults is commonly tested by means of same/different judgement tasks involving words and non-words and lexical decision tasks (see Chapters 1.2, 1.3 and 2.3). All the recognition tasks used in these studies, however, involve linguistic stimuli in isolation, so that we do not know whether there may be differences between recognition of items in isolation and in context. This limits our ability to predict the impact of recognition problems on the comprehension of fluent speech or continuous written language for both children and adults, as Morris (Chapter 1.3) points out (see also Tyler 1992), and on the acquisition process (see Morgan and Demuth 1996). The differences here are not so much between the child and adult fields as between clinicians and researchers, as most tests of recognition involve quite complex equipment that is not routinely available to clinicians. Although language impairment is at least as complex as physical illness, speech and language therapists, unlike physicians, are still expected to diagnose without the services of specialised laboratories!

Comprehension is tested mainly by means of matching or selection of pictures to words or sentences (see Chapters 2.2, 2.3, 3.2 and 3.3) or by judgements of semantic relatedness or opposition (see Chapters 2.2, 2.3, 3.2) and pragmatic appropriateness (see Chapters 4.2 and 4.3).

The production skills of children and adults are tested in exactly the same way with repetition (oral reproduction of auditory input) of words and sentences (see Chapters 1.2, 2.3, 3.2) and writing to dictation (written reproduction of auditory input) (see Chapters 1.2, 1.3, 3.2). There are also tasks – which I have termed 'silent production' – that involve processing pictures and then generating corresponding 'silent' phonology (see Chapter 2.2), or arranging written sentence fragments appropriately (see Chapters 3.2, 3.3). Methods of eliciting spontaneous, oral or written language are similar: pictures of single objects or actions have to be named (see Chapters 1.2, 1.3, 2.3), or descriptions of situations or events have to be provided (see Chapters 2.3, 3.2, 3.3). Both adults and children are asked to tell stories with or without pictures, and to engage in conversation either freely or within specified pragmatic contexts (see Chapters 4.2 and 4.3).

Measurement of performance on these tasks is always in terms of error rates supplemented with analyses of error types and error patterns. With both children and adults we still know very little about the timing of their performance, which limits our ability to build up a more dynamic picture of their psycholinguistic systems where the **rate of processing**, rather than the processing mechanisms or representations, might be a cause of impairment. This is mainly because language processing, a highly dynamic system, has been largely modelled in terms of static systems where timing has not been a central theoretical issue (but see Tyler 1992). Reducing dynamic systems to static ones is a convenient but misleading theoretical ploy that can make us lose sight of some crucial properties of systems.

From causes to remedies

Judging from the papers and the discussion at the conference, therapy is carried out with adults and children in remarkably similar ways. For both client groups it is not the task that distinguishes assessment from therapy. All the assessment tasks surveyed above are, or can be, used in therapy. For instance, the same auditory discrimination task is used in both assessment and therapy by Vance with a child and by Morris with an adult; Lewis and Speake (Chapter 2.2) use 'semantic links' judgements to assess and remediate Richard, and Best *et al.* (Chapter 2.3) use picture naming in both aspects of their work with JOW. What distinguishes therapy and assessment is how the client and the therapist **use** the task.

In therapy, the client's attention might be drawn to additional sources of information that can be tapped, or tapped more consistently and consciously, in performing the task, e.g. lip-reading in carrying out auditory discrimination (see Chapters 1.2 and 1.3).

Supporting or reinforcing cues can be provided at different points (see Chapters 1.2, 1.3, 2.3) affecting the client's use of information during the task. For instance, Best *et al.* (Chapter 2.3) suggest that the cueing aid JOW used in naming pictures during therapy

> ... explicitly required JOW to use partial orthographic knowledge to aid word finding, ... The aid, by requiring him to put these separate skills together, enabled him to make the link. (p. 122)

Different types of feedback can be given during the task in therapy (see for example Chapters 1.3 and 4.2), ranging from simply telling the client whether they are correct or not (Chapter 1.3) to more detailed discussion of the responses and the stimuli to be processed (see

Chapters 1.2, 3.2, 3.3, 4.2). It is striking that discussion and explanation take place as much with children as with adults.

Some therapies, however, involve more discussion and explanation than others. How do therapists decide whether to adopt a **minimalist** approach, with little intervention from the therapist apart from limited feedback, modelling or prompting, or an **interactive** method with detailed feedback to and from the client and explanation of what he or she is processing? If both approaches are adopted at different stages in the intervention (see Chapters 1.2 and 4.2), what motivates the selection of an approach for a particular stage? In none of the studies in this volume were such decisions made straightforwardly or automatically on the basis of the deficit alone.

A number of factors seem to influence the decisions with both children and adults, including the aim and focus of therapy, which may or may not overlap with the area of breakdown, the nature of the representations that are tapped during therapy, and the type of processing mechanisms involved. Minimalist approaches appear to be more common in two cases. First, when the representations involved are connected by arbitrary habitual association, e.g. lexical representations where the relation between the form (phonological or orthographic) of a word and its meaning is arbitrary and has to be learned through association. For instance, the aim of the therapy carried out by Best *et al.* (Chapter 2.3) with JOW was to improve his word retrieval for output. They focused on the representations involved in picture naming, a task that involves retrieving semantic representations arbitrarily associated to a phonological form. Their therapy approach was minimalist in that the therapist only intervened if JOW's response was incorrect and only by restricting his choice of letters on the cueing aid or by providing the target for him to repeat.

Secondly, a minimalist approach seems more likely to be adopted when the processing is automatic, unconscious or non-strategic, such as auditory perception or word-retrieval (see Chapters 1.2 and 1.3). Best *et al.* (Chapter 2.3), for example, say of their therapy that it has enabled JOW to make links between lexical representations and they add that

> This linking, however, is different in kind from the conscious and deliberate ways in which orthography has been used to improve word retrieval by, for instance, de Partz (1986) and Nickels (1992); instead the treatment has effected a fundamental change in the way JOW's word retrieval operates, altering automatic and not strategic processes in his linguistic system. (p. 122)

More interactive approaches, on the other hand, appear to be adopted when there is a systematic, rule-governed relationship between the representations the therapy focuses on, such as that between the plural or third person present marker and their various phonological realisations (see Chapter 1.2); or that between thematic roles and their realisation in particular positions in the sentence (see Chapters 3.2, 3.3).

Interactive forms of therapy also seem more likely when non-automatic, conscious and strategic processing is being targeted either because of the nature of the processing involved or to bypass 'normal' processes that are no longer available. Vance (Chapter 1.2), for example, talks about 'promoting phonological awareness skills', and Bryan (Chapter 3.2) defines the aim of therapy as 'to raise Gordon's awareness of the predicate argument structure of sentences to a conscious level'.

These are tentative suggestions. At the end of this conference, however, there can be no doubt that a greater theoretical understanding of what and how we assess and treat has benefited our work with adults and children.

Chapter 5.2
Psycholinguistic applications to language therapy

JANE MARSHALL

The conference 'Making New Connections' occurred at an interesting watershed in British speech and language therapy. In the paediatric field, the application of psycholinguistics to therapy was relatively new. This novelty engendered an enthusiasm and a belief that further applications would bring about significant progress in child language rehabilitation. In the adult domain, psycholinguistics, or **cognitive neuropsychology**, was much more established, and had already spawned numerous therapy studies (see for example Byng 1988, Nickels 1992, Riddoch and Humphreys 1994). This familiarity had, in turn, generated doubts. A number of commentators argued that cognitive neuropsychology left many crucial therapy questions unanswered, such as how to bring about changes in the language system (for example Caramazza 1989, Lesser and Milroy 1993). Some also made the point that therapies claiming to be based on a psycholinguistic theory of the deficit might equally have emerged from routine clinical observations. As a result, apparently psycholinguistic approaches might be difficult to distinguish from behaviourist drilling.

On a broader field, aphasia therapy was seeing the beginning of a more general debate about the whole purpose of rehabilitation. Drawing upon ideas within the disability movement, some clinicians questioned the traditional focus of therapy on the language impairment. While not dismissing such impairment centred work, there was a call for novel forms of therapy which could identify and challenge the barriers which society and disabling environments impose upon the aphasic individual (Parr *et al.* 1995, Pound 1996).

In the light of these different ideas about rehabilitation it might be useful to reflect upon what psycholinguistics can, and cannot, bring to language therapy and to acknowledge some of the potential misapplications of the approach. In so doing, we will return to some of the broad issues raised in our introduction.

The first obvious application of psycholinguistics is in identifying the language deficit and, just as importantly, any intact language skills. Without models of language processing, we are necessarily limited to behavioural observations about our patients and the people they interact with. For example, we might observe that communication breaks down mainly because of an anomia. In addition, we might begin to uncover environmental factors which exacerbate the anomia and detect problem solving strategies that the person, or his or her communication partners, can bring to bear. Such observations remain a crucial component of our initial investigations. However, with the advent of psycholinguistics we can formulate more specific hypotheses about the processing limitations which give rise to the problem. For example, we might note that the person can describe or gesture objects which he or she cannot name. This suggests that some semantic skills are available and that the problem may therefore reside at the phonological level.

These psycholinguistic hypotheses give assessment a new direction. Rather than assessing exhaustively from scratch, the clinician can select specific measures with which to pursue early hunches. Thus, in the case of a naming problem, the hypothesis that semantics is intact can be assessed using a number of tasks which require the person to access meaning, either from words or pictures. If the person succeeds on these tasks we can be relatively confident that semantic information is available, at least to some degree. Similarly, we might investigate whether the person can access lexical phonologies, e.g. by comparing naming with reading aloud and repetition and by exploring the effects of cues. Such tasks can indicate whether the problem affects the phonological representations themselves, or simply access to them.

Psycholinguistically driven assessment has a number of potential advantages over other approaches. If applied properly, it can also avoid the danger of over-testing. Instead of exploring every language skill, e.g. through an extended language battery, the clinician focuses on those skills which are most relevant to the person's key problem and its potential treatment. The results of such assessments should also be relatively easy to interpret, mainly because they were administered with a specific question in mind.

In the developmental domain, psycholinguistic assessment provides an essential complement to assessments based on profiles of normal language development. Such profiles are useful for identifying delay and for highlighting particular areas of difficulty. However, they often tell us very little about the exact nature of the problem. One difficulty here is the typical unevenness of the profile. In other words, the child may deal with some aspects of language relatively well, but not others. Such discrepancies call for a hypothesis about which processing skills are intact and which are impaired. This, in turn, can act as a springboard to further psycholinguistic investigation.

The main purpose of psycholinguistic theory is to provide guidance for therapy. Here it is important not to overstate the case. Several commentators have rightly argued that the psycholinguistic analysis does not directly prescribe the treatment (Caramazza 1989, Byng *et al.* 1990, Hillis 1993). This is partly because psycholinguistic theories do not themselves grapple with issues of therapy, such as which treatments work for which deficits, and how treatment affects the language system (if at all). Such questions about therapy constitute a whole new theoretical domain which has only recently been opened up (e.g. Byng 1995).

Given our current state of knowledge, there are a number of contributions that psycholinguistics can make to therapy. Perhaps the main one is in helping us to identify a target for intervention, and, in particular, a target which is more specified than a mere statement of the behaviour that we hope to achieve. For example, in a case of anomia, we do not need an extensive psycholinguistic analysis to know that improving word finding would be a good idea. Yet a psycholinguistic therapy hypothesis will elaborate upon that aim. It will specify the type of processing that we hope to encourage and how that processing might bring about the desired increase in production. Such a hypothesis has a number of advantages. First of all, it helps us to be more specific about the aims of therapy with our patients and their relatives. Secondly, it provides pointers to the content of therapy, not solely in terms of tasks but also in terms of the interactions that occur during those tasks. For example, if our aim is to boost semantic processing we are likely to use semantic tasks, such as 'odd one out' tasks or word-to-picture matching. However, we might also invite the person to think about what meanings are available for certain words (i.e. by gesturing possible associations) and to introspect about how he or she arrived at those meanings. This potentially introduces a metalinguistic component to therapy, in which the person is encouraged to reflect upon the processing that they apply in any particular language task and to manipulate that processing in a conscious manner.

We would therefore argue that psycholinguistically based intervention opens up a new form of partnership between the therapist and patient. Construed in this way, it is not an approach which simply aims to lessen the impairment, with the patient as a relatively passive participant in the process. Rather, it seeks to give patients more insight into their processing and hence more control over it. Of course, not all therapy takes this form. As Maria Black suggests in Chapter 5.1, there is also a place for 'minimalist' therapy, which involves comparatively little conscious reflection and where the aim is simply to practise, and hence strengthen, automatic on-line processes.

One further contribution that psycholinguistics can make is in guiding evaluation. Such evaluation sets out not only to explore changes in surface language behaviours, but also to explore whether those changes are a consequence of improved or adapted processing. For example, we might evaluate a 'semantic naming programme' partly by assessing word finding before and after therapy, but also by probing for changes in semantic skills. The latter may well call upon assessments which have little to do with naming *per se*, such as comprehension or even non-verbal tasks. Evaluation should also investigate whether any apparent processing changes have brought about improvements in the person's daily communication. Such 'functional' evaluation has typically been seen as somehow beyond the psycholinguistic domain. Yet we fail to see why. Therapy may well promote processing skills which can be marshalled in the supportive clinical environment, but not in the cut and thrust of normal interactions. Disparities between formal assessment and more naturalistic, conversational performance provide further insights into the changes which may have taken place, as well as alerting the clinician to work that still needs to be done.

In this section, we have discussed the potential contribution of psycholinguistics to language therapy. The realisation of that potential depends on the active and continued exploration of how aspects of language processing interact and how intervention in one aspect can affect another. Having identified the potential of this approach, it is important to acknowledge its dangers. One of the main dangers, we believe, is that it is all too easy to become fixated with the hypothesised site of the language deficit and make that the focus of therapy. This approach compromises the overall picture of how the individual processes language and communicates with other people and inevitably leads to rather detached, functionally irrelevant programmes.

Applied properly, psycholinguistic intervention seeks to identify the site of the deficit but recognises that this may not be the focus of therapy. One alternative is to turn our attention to strengths within the system which can overcome or circumvent the deficit. Another is to direct our attention to the person's environment. This is where psycholinguistics can complement ideas emerging from the disability movement. These ideas argue that much of the disability experienced by the individual is created by the disabling environment. Therefore the efforts of rehabilitation teams should be directed towards identifying and removing the barriers which bar social access. An obvious example of such barrier removal, in the context of physical disability, is the provision of ramps in public buildings. Yet in the context of aphasia, barrier removal is necessarily more subtle. This is because what constitutes a barrier will partly depend upon the specific difficulties of the individual and, similarly, the removal of barriers on their particular skills. For example, a person with a severe deficit in auditory discrimination will encounter major barriers in certain conversational settings. These barriers might be lowered if the conversational partners adopt a number of strategies, such as providing a strong semantic context for new information, which enables the aphasic person to bring his or her skills to bear. Thus a sound understanding of the person's processing strengths and weaknesses is an essential starting point even for this type of intervention.

Finally, we would argue that understanding the deficit provides insight into the inevitable internal conflicts which arise from a language disorder. Take the child who has so much to say, but no means of saying it, or the adult who once accessed language automatically, but now struggles for the most mundane words. Those of us who do not share the experience can never fully understand the personal implications of a language disorder. However, we can at least explore the problem with the individual and thus show our respect for their dilemma. One such exploration is conducted through psycholinguistics.

References

Aitchison, J. (1987). Words in the Mind: An Introduction to the Mental Lexicon. Oxford: Blackwell.

Allport, D.A. (1985). Distributed memory, modular subsystems and dysphasia. In S.K. Newman and R. Epstein (eds.), Current Perspectives in Dysphasia. Edinburgh: Churchill Livingstone.

Amery, J.S. and Cartright, S. (1989). First 1,000 Word Book. London: Usborn.

Atkinson, M. (1979). Pre-requisites for reference. In E. Ochs and B. Schieffelin (eds.), Developmental Pragmatics. New York: Academic Press.

Badecker, W. and Caramazza, A. (1985). On considerations of method and theory governing the use of clinical categories in neurolinguistics and cognitive neuropsychology: The case against agrammatism. Cognition, 20, 97–125.

Baker, E., Blumstein, S.E. and Goodglass, H. (1981). Interaction between phonological and semantic factors in auditory comprehension. Neuropsychologia, 19, 1–15.

Baron-Cohen, S., Leslie, A.M. and Frith, U. (1985). Does the autistic child have a 'theory of mind'. Cognition, 21, 37–46.

Barry, C., Morrison, C.M. and Ellis, A.W. (in press). Naming the Snodgrass and Vanderwart pictures: effects of age of acquisition, frequency and name agreement. Quarterly Journal of Experimental Psychology.

Bear, D. (1983). Hemispheric specialization and the neurology of emotion. Archives of Neurology, 40, 195–202.

Beer, S. (1996). It's the Beer talking. New Times, No.114, 12.

Behrmann, M. and Byng, S. (1993). A cognitive approach to the neurorehabilitation of acquired language disorders. In D.I. Margolin (eds.), Cognitive Neuropsychology in Clinical Practice, pp. 327–50. New York: Oxford University Press.

Berman, M. and Peelle, L.M. (1967). Self-generated cues: a method for aiding aphasic and apraxic patients. Journal of Speech and Hearing Disorders, 32, 372–6.

Berndt, R (1987). Symptom co-occurrence and dissociation in the interpretation of agrammatism. In M. Coltheart, G. Sartori and R. Job (eds.), The Cognitive Neuropsychology of Language. Hillsdale, NJ: Erlbaum.

Best, W. (1996). When racquets are baskets but baskets are biscuits, where do the words come from: a single case study of formal paraphasic errors in aphasia. Cognitive Neuropsychology, 13, 443–80.

Best, W., Howard, D., Bruce, C. and Gatehouse, C. (in press). Cueing the words: a single case study of treatments for anomia. Neuropsychological Rehabilitation.

Bever, T.G. (1992). The demons and the beast–modular and nodular kinds of knowledge. In R.G.Reilly and N.E. Sharkey (eds.), Connectionist Approaches to Natural Language Processing, pp. 213–53. Hove, Sussex: Erlbaum.

Bigland, S. and Speake, J. (1992). Semantic Links. Ponteland: STASS Publications.

Bishop, D.V.M. (1982a). Test for Reception of Grammar. London: Medical Research Council.

Bishop, D.V.M. (1982b). Comprehension of spoken, written and signed sentences in childhood language disorders. Journal of Child Psychology and Psychiatry, 23, 1–20.

Bishop, D.V.M. and Adams, C. (1989). Conversational characteristics of children with semantic pragmatic disorder II: what features lead to a judgement of inappropriacy? British Journal of Disorders of Communication, 24, 241–63.

Black, M., Nickels, L. and Byng, S. (1992). Patterns of sentence processing deficit: processing simple sentences can be a complex matter. Journal of Neurolinguistics, 6, 79–101.

Blank, M., Gessner, M. and Esposito, A. (1979). Language without communication: a case study. Journal of Child Language, 6, 329–52.

Borod, J., Koff, E., Lorch, M. and Nicholas, M. (1986). The expression and perception of facial emotion in brain-damaged patients. Neuropsychologia, 24, 169–80.

Brett, L., Chiat, S. and Pilcher, C. (1988). Stages and units in output processing: some evidence from voicing and fronting processes in children. Language and Cognitive Processes, 2, 165–177.

Bridgeman, E. and Snowling, M. (1988). The perception of phoneme sequence: a comparison of dyspraxic and normal children. British Journal of Disorders of Communication, 23, 245–52.

Brinton, B. and Fujiki, M. (1982). A comparison of request-response sequences in the discourse of normal and language impaired children. Journal of Speech and Hearing Research, 47, 57–62.

Broca, P. (1865). Sur le siège de la faculté du langage articulé. Bulletin d'Anthropologie 6, 377–93.

Brownell, H., Michel, D., Powelson, J. and Gardner, H. (1983). Suprise but not coherence: sensitivity to verbal humor in right-hemisphere patients. Brain and Language, 18, 20–7.

Bruce, C. and Howard, D. (1987). Computer generated cues: an effective aid for naming in aphasia. British Journal of Disorders of Communication, 22, 191–201.

Bryan, A. and Howard, D. (1992). Frozen phonology thawed: the analysis and remediation of a developmental disorder of real word phonology. European Journal of Disorders of Communication, 27, 343–65.

Bryan, K. (1988). Assessment of language disorders after right hemisphere damage. British Journal of Disorders of Communication, 23, 111–27.

Bryan, K. (1989). Language prosody and the right hemisphere. Aphasiology, 3, 285–99.

Bryan, K. (1994). The Right Hemisphere Language Battery. London: Whurr.

Butterworth, B. (1979). Hesitation and the production of verbal paraphasias and neologisms in jargon aphasia. Brain and Language, 8, 133–61.

Butterworth, B. (1980). Some constraints on models of language production. In B. Butterworth (eds.), Language production, Vol 1. London: Academic Press.

Butterworth, B. (1985). Jargon aphasia: processes and strategies. In S. Newman and R. Epstein (eds.), Current Perspectives in Dysphasia. Edinburgh: Churchill, Livingstone.

Butterworth, B.L. (1989). Lexical access in speech production. In W. Marslen-Wilson (eds.), Lexical Representation and Process. Cambridge, MA: MIT Press.

Butterworth, B. (1992). Disorders of phonological encoding. Cognition 42, 261–86.

Butterworth, B.L., Howard, D. and McLoughlin, P.J. (1984). The semantic deficit in aphasia: the relationship between semantic errors in auditory comprehension and picture naming. Neuropsychologia, 22, 409–26.

Byng, S. (1988). Sentence processing deficits: theory and therapy. Cognitive Neuropsychology, 5, 629–76.

Byng, S. (1995). What is aphasia therapy? In C. Code and D. Muller (eds.), Treatment of Aphasia: from Theory to Practice. London: Whurr.

Byng, S. and Black, M. (1995). What makes a therapy? Some parameters of therapeutic intervention in aphasia. European Journal of Disorders of Communication, 30, 303–16.

Byng, S. and Coltheart, M. (1986). Aphasia therapy research: Methodological requirements and illustrative results. In E. Hjelmquist and L.G.Nilsson (eds.), Communication and Handicap. Amsterdam: Elsevier.

Byng, S., Kay, J., Edmundson, A. and Scott, C. (1990). Aphasia tests reconsidered. Aphasiology, 4, 67–91.

Byng, S., Nickels, L. and Black, M. (1994). Replicating therapy for mapping deficits in agrammatism: remapping the deficit? Aphasiology, 8, 315–41.

Caramazza, A. (1985). The logic of neuropsychological research and the problem of patient classification in aphasia. Brain and Language, 21, 9–20.

Caramazza, A. (1989). Cognitive neuropsychology and rehabilitation: an unfulfilled promise. In X. Seron and G. Deloche (eds.), Cognitive Approaches in Neuropsychological Rehabilitation. Hillsdale, NJ: Erlbaum.

Caramazza, A. and Hillis, A.E. (1993). For a theory of rehabilitation. Neuropsychological Rehabilitation, 3, 217–34.

Caramazza, A., Berndt, R.S. and Basili, A.G. (1983). The selective impairment of phonological processing: a case study. Brain and Language, 18, 128–74.

Caramazza, A., Hillis, A., Rapp, C. and Romani, C. (1990). The multiple semantics hypothesis multiple confusions. Cognitive Neuropsychology, 7, 161–89.

Chiat, S. (1983). Why *Mikey's* right and *my key's* wrong: the significance of stress and word boundaries in a child's output system. Cognition, 14, 275–300.

Chiat, S. (1994). From lexical access to lexical output: what is the problem for children with impaired phonology? In M. Yavas (eds.), First and Second Language phonology. San Diego: Singular Publishing Group.

Chiat. S. and Hunt, J. (1993). Connections between phonology and semantics: an exploration of lexical processing in a language impaired child. Child Language, Teaching and Therapy, 9, 200–13.

Chieffi, S., Carlomagno, S., Silveri, M. and Gainotti G. (1989). The influence of semantic and perceptual factors on lexical comprehension in aphasic and right brain-damaged patients. Cortex, 25, 591–8.

Coltheart, M. (1980). Analysing acquired disorders of reading. Unpublished manuscript: Birkbeck College.

Coltheart, M. and Byng, S. (1989). A treatment for surface dyslexia. In X. Seron and G. Deloche (eds.), Cognitive Approaches in Neuropsychological Rehabilitation. Hillsdale, NJ: Erlbaum.

Coltheart, M., Bates, A. and Castles, A. (1994). Cognitive neuropsychology and rehabilitation. In M.J. Riddoch and G.W. Humphreys (eds.), Cognitive Neuropsychology and Cognitive Rehabilitation. Hove, Sussex: Erlbaum.

Conti-Ramsden, G. and Gunn, M. (1986). The development of conversational disability: a case study. British Journal of Disorders of Communication, 21, 339–51.

Craig, H.K. and Evans, T.M. (1989). Turn exchange characteristics of SLI children's simultaneous and nonsimultaneous speech. Journal of Speech and Hearing Disorders, 54, 334–47.

Craig, H.K. and Gallagher, T.M. (1979). The structural characteristics of monologues in the speech of normal children: syntactic non-conversational aspects. Journal of Speech and Hearing Research, 22, 46–62.

Crystal, D., Fletcher, P. and Garman, M. (1982). The Grammatical Analysis of Language Disability: A Procedure for Assessment and Remediation (revised edn). London : Edward Arnold.

De Partz, M-P. (1986). Reeducation of a deep dyslexic patient: rationale of the method and results. Cognitive Neuropsychology, 3, 149–77.

De Wijngaert, E. and Gommers, K. (1993). Language rehabilitation in the Landau-Kleffner syndrome: considerations and approaches. Aphasiology, 7, 475–80.

Dean, E.C. and Howell, J. (1986). Developing linguistic awareness: a theoretically based approach to phonological disorders. British Journal of Disorders of Communication, 21, 223–38.

Dean, E.C., Howell, J., Waters, D. and Reid, J. (1995). Metaphon: a metalinguistic approach to the treatment of phonological disorder in children. Clinical Linguistics and Phonetics, 9, 1–19.

Dell, G.S. (1986). A spreading activation theory of retrieval in sentence production. Psychological Review, 93, 283–321.

Dell, G. (1988). The retrieval of phonological forms in production: test of predictions from a connectionist model. Journal of Memory and Language, 27, 124–42.

Dell, G.S. (1989). The retrieval of phonological forms in production: tests of predictions from a connectionist model. In W. Marslen-Wilson (eds.), Lexical Representation and Process. Cambridge, MA: MIT Press.

Denes, G. and Semenza, C. (1975). Auditory modality-specific anomia: evidence from a case of pure word deafness. Cortex, 11, 401–11.

Denes, G., Balleillo, S., Volterra, V. and Pelligrini, A. (1986). Oral and written language in a case of childhood phonemic deafness. Brain and Language, 29, 252–67.

Donahue, M., Pearl, R. and Bryan, T. (1980). Learning disabled children's conversational competence: responses to inadequate messages. Applied Psycholinguistics, 1, 387–403.

Dugas, M. and Moreau, N. (1972). Agnosie auditive congenitale. Reéducation orthophonique, 68, 211–20.

Dunn, L.M., Whetton, C. and Pintilie, D. (1982). British Picture Vocabulary Scales. Windsor: NFER Nelson.

Eisenson, J. (1962). Language and intellectual modifications associated with right cerebral damage. Language and Speech, 5, 49–53.

Ellis, A.W. (1985). The production of spoken words: a cognitive neuropsychological perspective. In A.W. Ellis (eds.), Progress in the Psychology of Language: Vol. 2. London: Erlbaum.

Ellis, A.W. and Young, A.W. (1988). Human Cognitive Neuropsychology. London: Erlbaum.

Ervin-Tripp, S. (1977). Wait for me, roller skate. In S. Ervin-Tripp and C. Mitchell-Kernan (eds.), Child Discourse. New York: Academic Press.

Farah, M.J. and McClelland, J.L. (1991). A computational model of semantic memory impairment: modality-specificity and emergent category-specificity. Journal of Experimental Psychology: General, 120, 339–57.

Ferry, P.C. and Cooper, J.A. (1978). Sign language in communication disorders. Journal of Pediatrics, 90, 547–52.

Fey, M.E. and Leonard, L.B. (1983). Pragmatic skills of children with specific language impairment. In T.M. Gallagher and C.A. Prutting (eds.), Pragmatic Assessment and Intervention Issues in Language. San Diego: College Hill Press.

Fisher, C., Hall, G., Rakowitz, S. and Gleitman, L. (1994). When is it better to receive than to give: syntactic and conceptual constraints on vocabulary growth. Lingua, 92, 333–75.

Forster, K.I. (1976). Accessing the mental lexicon. In R.J. Wales and E. Walker (eds.), New Approaches to Language Mechanisms. Amsterdam: North-Holland.

Franklin, S. (1989). Dissociations in auditory word comprehension: evidence from nine fluent aphasic patients. Aphasiology, 3, 189–207.

Franklin, S., Turner, J.E. and Ellis, A.W. (1992). ADA Comprehension Battery. Available from Action for Dysphasic Adults, Canterbury House, Royal Street, London SE1 7LL.

Franklin, S., Howard, D. and Patterson, K. (1995). Abstract word anomia. Cognitive Neuropsychology, 12, 549–66.

Frith, U. (1989). A new look at language and communication in autism. British Journal of Disorders of Communication, 24, 123–51.

Gainotti, G., Caltagirone, C. and Miceli, G. (1983). Selective impairment of semantic-lexical discrimination in right brain-damaged patients. In E. Perecman (eds.), Cognitive Processing in the Right Hemisphere. Orlando, FL: Academic Press.

Gallagher, T. (eds.), (1991) Pragmatics of Language: Clinical Practice Issues. London: Chapman & Hall.

Gallagher, T.M. and Darnton, B.A. (1978). Conversational aspects of the speech of language impaired children: revision behaviours. Journal of Speech and Hearing Research, 21, 118–35.

Garrett, M. (1988). Processes in language production. In F. Newmeyer (eds.), Linguistics: The Cambridge Survey, Vol 3. Cambridge: Cambridge University Press.

Garrett, M.F. (1980). Levels of speech processing in sentence production. In B. Butterworth (eds.), Language Production, Vol. 1: Speech and Talk. London: Academic Press.

Gerard, C.L., Dugas, M. and Sagar, D. (1991). Speech therapy in Landau and Kleffner syndrome. In I.P. Martins et al. (eds.), Acquired Aphasia in Children: Acquisition and Breakdown of Language in the Developing Brain, pp. 279–90. Dordrecht: Kluwer.

Gielewski, E. (1989). Acoustic analysis and auditory retraining in the remediation of sensory aphasia. In C. Code and D.J. Muller (eds.), Aphasia Therapy, pp 138–45. London: Whurr.

Green, E. and Barber, P. (1981). An auditory stroop effect with judgements of speaker gender. Perception and Psychophysics, 30, 459–66.

Greenlee, M. (1981). Learning to tell the forest from the trees: unravelling discourse features of a psychotic child. First Language, 2, 83–102.

Grice, H. (1975). Logic and conversation. In Cole, P. and Morgan, J. (eds.), Syntax and Semantics, Vol. 3: Speech Acts. New York: Academic Press.

Guilford, J. (1967). The Nature of Human Intelligence. New York: McGraw-Hill.

Haegeman, L. (1991). Introduction to Government and Binding Theory. Oxford: Blackwell.

Halliday, M.A.K. (1975). Learning How To Mean: Explorations in the Development of Language. London: Edward Arnold.

Happe, F. (1991). Theory of mind and communication in autism. Unpublished PhD thesis, University of London.

Harding, D. (1993). Using word initial graphemes to facilitate spoken naming:an investigation of self-cueing in an aphasic individual. Unpublished MSc thesis, Birkbeck College, London.

Harley, T.A. and MacAndrew, S.B.G. (1992). Modelling paraphasias in normal and aphasic speech. Proceedings of the 14th Annual Conference of the Cognitive Science Society, Bloomington, IN, pp. 378–83.

Haynes, C. (1992). Vocabulary deficit – one problem or many? Child Language Teaching and Therapy, 8(1), 1–17.

Heilman, K., Scholes, R. and Watson, R. (1975). Auditory affective agnosia. Journal of Neurology, Neurosurgery and Psychiatry, 38, 69–72.

Hewlett, N. (1990). Processes of development and production. In P. Grunwell (eds.), Developmental Speech Disorders. Edinburgh: Churchill Livingstone.

Hillis, A.E. (1989). Efficacy and generalisation of treatment for aphasic naming errors. Archives of Physical Medicine and Rehabilitation, 70, 632–6.

Hillis, A. (1993). The role of models of language processing in rehabilitation of language impairments. Aphasiology, 7, 5–26.

Hillis, A. and Caramazza, A. (1994). Theories of lexical processing and rehabilitation of lexical deficits. In M.J. Riddoch and G.W. Humphreys (eds.), Cognitive Neuropsychology and Cognitive Rehabilitation. Hove, Sussex: Erlbaum.

Hillis, A.E. and Caramazza, A. (1995). Converging evidence for the interaction of semantic and sublexical phonological information in accessing lexical representations for spoken output. Cognitive Neuropsychology, 12, 187–227.

Hirsh-Pasek, K., Tucker, M. and Michnick Golinkoff, R. (1996). Dynamic systems theory: reinterpreting 'prosodic bootstrapping' and its role in language acquisition. In J.L. Morgan and K. Demuth (eds.), Signal to Syntax, pp. 439–66. Mahwah, NJ: Erlbaum.

Hobson, P. (1993). Autism and the Development of Mind. Hove, Sussex: Erlbaum.

Hodges, J. (1994). Cognitive Assessment for Clinicians. Oxford: Oxford University Press.

Hodson, B.W. and Paden, E.P. (1983). Targeting Remedial Speech: A phonological Approach to Remediation. San Diego, CA: College-Hill Press.

Howard, D. and Franklin, S. (1990). Memory without rehearsal. In T. Shallice and G. Vallar (eds.), Neuropsychological Impairments of Short-Term Memory. Cambridge: Cambridge University Press.

Howard, D. and Hatfield, F.M. (1987). Aphasia Therapy: Historical and Contemporary Issues. London: Erlbaum.

Howard, D. and Orchard-Lisle, V. (1984). On the origin of semantic errors in naming: evidence from the case of a global aphasic. Cognitive Neuropsychology, 1, 163–90.

Howard, D. and Patterson, K.E. (1992). Pyramids and Palm Trees. Bury St Edmunds: Thames Valley Test Company.

Howard, D., Best, W., Bruce, C. and Gatehouse, C. (1995). Operativity and animacy effects in aphasic naming. European Journal of Disorders of Communication, 30, 286–302.

Howard, D., Patterson, K., Franklins, S., Orchard-Lisle, V. and Morton, J. (1985a) The facilitation of picture naming in aphasia. Cognitive Neuropsychology, 2, 49–80.

Howard, D., Patterson, K., Franklins, S., Orchard-Lisle, V. and Morton, J. (1985b) The treatment of word retrieval deficits in aphasia: a comparison of two therapy methods. Brain, 108, 817–829.

Huskisson, J.A. (1973). Acquired receptive language difficulty in childhood. British Journal of Disorders of Communication, 8, 54–63.

Hyde-Wright, S. and Cray, B. (1990). A teacher's and a speech therapist's approach to management. In K. Mogford-Bevan and J. Saddler (eds.), Child Language

Disability, Vol II: Semantic and Pragmatic Difficulties. Multi Lingual Matters, Language Through Reading. Invalid Children's Aid Association.

Joanette, Y., Goulet, P., Ska, B. and Nespoulous, J-L. (1986). Informative content of narrative discourse in right-brain-damaged right-handers. Brain and Language, 29, 81–105.

Jones, E.V. (1984). Word order processing in aphasia: effect of verb semantics. In F.C. Rose (ed.), Advances in Neurology, 42. Progress in Aphasiology. New York: Raven Press

Jones, E.V. (1986). Building the foundations for sentence production in a non-fluent aphasic. British Disorders of Communication, 21, 63–82.

Jones, E.V. (1989). A year in the life of EVJ and PC. Proceedings of the Summer Conference of the British Aphasiology Society. Cambridge, June 1989.

Jones, S., Smedley, M. and Jennings, M. (1986). Case study: a child with high level language disorder characterised by syntactic, semantic and pragmatic difficulties. In Advances in Working with Language Disordered Children. ICAN.

Kay, J., Lesser, R. and Coltheart, M. (1992). PALPA, Psycholinguistic Assessments of Language Processing in Aphasia. Hove, Sussex: Erlbaum.

Keenan, E. and Schieffelin, B. (1976). Topic as a discourse notion: a study of topic in the conversation of children and adults. In C. Li (eds.), Subject and Topic. New York: Academic Press.

Kimura, D. (1967). Functional asymmetry of the brain in dichotic listening. Cortex, 3, 163–78.

Kintsch, W. and van Dijk, T. (1978). Toward a model of text comprehension and production. Psychological Review, 85, 363–94.

LeDorze, G., Boulay, N., Gaudreau, J. and Brassard (1994). The contrasting effects of a semantic versus a formal-semantic technique for the facilitation of naming in a case of anomia. Aphasiology, 8, 127–41.

Lees, J. (1993). Children with Acquired Aphasias. London: Whurr.

Lesser, R. (1974). Verbal comprehension in aphasia: an English version of three Italian tests. Cortex, 10, 247–63.

Lesser, R. and Algar, L. (1995). Towards combining the cognitive neuropsychological and pragmatic in aphasia therapy. Neuropsychological Rehabilitation, 5, 67–92.

Lesser, R. and Milroy, L. (1993). Linguistics and Aphasia: Psycholinguistic and Pragmatic Aspects of Intervention. London: Longman.

Levelt, W.J.M. (1989). Speaking: From Intention to Articulation. Cambridge, MA: MIT Press.

Levelt, W.J.M. (1992) Accessing words in speech production. Cognition, 42, 1–22.

Levy, J. (1974). Psychological implications of bilateral asymmetry. In S.J. Diamond and J. Beaumont (eds.), Hemisphere Functions in the Human Brain. London: Elek Science.

Lewis, S. (1994). The jigsaw of lexical development–how do the pieces fit together in children aged five, six and seven? Unpublished MSc Dissertation, NHCSS, London.

Lewis, S. and Bird, T. (1995). Talking Semantics. Totness, BirdArt.

Lewis, S. and Papier, T. (1996). Talking Phonology. Unpublished, Totness, BirdArt.

Locke, J. (1980). The inference of speech perception in the phonologically disordered child. Part 2: some clinically novel procedures, their use, some findings. Journal of Speech and Hearing Disorders, 45, 445–68.

Luria, A.R. (1970). Traumatic Aphasia. The Hague: Mouton.

MacDonald, S. (1993). Viewing the brain sideways? Frontal versus right hemisphere explanations of non-aphasic language disorders. Aphasiology, 7, 535–49.

Mackay, D. and Thompson, B. (1970). Breakthrough to Literacy. London: Longman.

McCarthy, R. and Warrington, E. (1985). Category specificity in an agrammatic patient: the relative impairment of verb retrieval and comprehension. Neuropsychologia, 23, 709–27.

McTear, M.F. (1985a). Children's Conversation. Oxford: Blackwell.

McTear, M. (1985b). Pragmatic disorders: a question of direction. European Journal of Disorders of Communication, 20, 119–27.

McTear, M.F. (1990). Is there such a thing as conversational disability? In K. Mogford-Bevan and J. Saddler (eds.), Child Language Disability Vol II: Semantic and Pragmatic Difficulties. Multi Lingual Matters.

McTear, M. and Conti-Ramsden, G. (1992). Pragmatic Disability in Children. London: Whurr.

Mandler, J. and Johnson, N. (1977). Remembrance of things parsed: story structure and recall. Cognitive Psychology, 9, 111–51.

Marshall, J. (1994). Sentence processing in aphasia: single case treatment studies. Unpublished Ph.D thesis, City University, London.

Marshall, J. (1995). The mapping hypothesis and aphasia therapy. Aphasiology, 9, 517–39.

Marshall, J., Pound, C., White-Thomson, M. and Pring, T. (1990). The use of picture/word matching tasks to assist word retrieval in aphasic patients. Aphasiology, 4, 167–84.

Marshall, J., Pring, T. and Chiat, S. (1993). Sentence processing therapy: working at the level of the event. Aphasiology, 7, 177–99.

Marshall, J., Pring, T., Chiat, S. and Robson, J. (1996). Calling a salad a federation: an investigation of semantic jargon, 1, nouns. Journal of Neurolinguistics,9, 237–50.

Martin, N., Dell, G.S., Saffran, E.M. and Schwartz, M.F. (1994). Origins of paraphasias in deep dysphasia: testing the consequences of a decay impairment to an interactive spreading activation account of lexical retrieval. Brain and Language, 47, 609–60.

Martin, N., Gagnon, D.A., Schwartz, M.F., Dell, G.S. and Saffran, E.M. (1996). Phonological facilitation of semantic errors in normal and aphasic speakers. Language and Cognitive Processes 11(3), 257–82.

Martin, R. and Blossom Stach, C. (1986). Evidence of syntactic deficit in a fluent aphasic. Brain and Language, 28, 196–234.

Masterson, J., Hazan, V. and Wijayatilake, L. (1995). Phonemic processing problems in developmental phonological dyslexia. Cognitive Neuropsychology, 12, 233–59.

Menn, L. (1983). Development of articulatory, phonetic, and phonological capabilities. In B. Butterworth (eds.), Language production, Vol 2. London: Academic Press.

Menn, L. and Matthei, E. (1992). The 'two-lexicon' account of child phonology: looking back, looking ahead. In C.A. Ferguson, L. Menn, C. Stoel-Gammon (eds.), Phonological development: models, research, implications. Timonium, MD: York Press.

Miceli, G., Mazzucchi, A., Menn, L. and Goodglass, H. (1983). Contrasting cases of agrammatic aphasia without comprehension disorder. Brain and Language, 19, 65–97.

Miceli, G., Amitrano, A., Capasso, R. and Caramazza, A. (1994). The remediation of anomia resulting from output lexical damage: analysis of two cases. Manuscript submitted for publication.

Milroy, L. (1988). Profile for analysing conversational disability. Unpublished manuscript, Department of Speech, University of Newcastle upon Tyne.

Mitchum, C. and Berndt, R. (1994). Verb retrieval and sentence construction: effects of targeted intervention. In M. Riddoch and G. Humphreys (eds.), Cognitive Neuropsychology and Cognitive Rehabilitation. Hove: Erlbaum.

Monsell, S. (1987). On the relation between lexical input and output pathways for speech. In A. Alport, D. Mackay, W. Prinz and E. Scheerer (eds.), Language Perception and Production: Relationships between Listening, Speaking, Reading and Writing. London: Academic Press.

Morgan, J.L. and Demuth, K. (eds.). (1996). Signal to Syntax. Mahwah, NJ: Erlbaum.

Morgan-Barry, R. (1988). The Auditory Discrimination and Attention Test. Windsor: NFER-Nelson.

Morris, J., Franklin, S., Ellis, A.W., Turner, J. and Bailey, P.J. (1996). Remediating a speech perception deficit in an aphasic patient. Aphasiology, 10, 137–58.

Morrison, C., Ellis, A. and Quinlan, P. (1992). Age of acquisition, not word frequency, affects object naming, not object recognition. Memory and Cognition, 20, 705–14.

Myers, P. (1994). Communcation disorders associated with right-hemisphere brain damage. In R. Chapey (eds.), Language Intervention Strategies in Adult Aphasia. Baltimore: Williams and Wilkins.

Naeser, M.A., Hass, G., Mazurski, P. and Laughlin, S. (1986). Sentence level auditory comprehension treatment program for aphasic adults. Archives of Physical Medicine and Rehabilitation, 67, 393–9.

Nettleton, J. and Lesser, R. (1991). Therapy for naming difficulties in aphasia: application of a cognitive neuropsychological model. Journal of Neurolinguistics, 6, 139–57.

Nickels, L.A. (1992). The autocue? Self-generated phonemic cues in the treatment of a disorder of reading and naming. Cognitive Neuropsychology, 9, 155–82.

Nickels, L.A. and Best, W. (1996a). Therapy for naming deficits: specifics, surprises and suggestions. Aphasiology, 10, 21–47.

Nickels, L.A. and Best, W. (1996b). Therapy for naming deficits: principles, puzzles and progress. Aphasiology, 10, 109–36.

Norman, D. and Shallice, T. (1980). Attention to action: willed and automatic control of behaviour. In R. Davidson, G. Schwartz and D. Shapiro (eds.), Consciousness and Self-Regulation. Advances in Research and Theory. New York: Plenum.

Parr, S., Pound, C. and Marshall, J. (1995). A handful of power for aphasic people. Bulletin of the College of Speech and Language Therapists, Issue 517.

Passy, J. (1990). Cued articulation. Ponteland: STASS Publications.

Patterson, K.E. and Shewell, C. (1987). Speak and spell: dissociations and word-class effects. In M. Coltheart, R. Job and G. Sartori (eds.), The cognitive neuropsychology of language. Hillsdale, NJ: Erlbaum.

Perkins, M., Body, R. and Parker, M. (1995). Closed head injury: assessment and remediation of topic bias and repetitiveness. In M. Perkins and S. Howard (eds.), Case Studies in Clinical Linguistics. London: Whurr.

Pinker, S. (1989). Learnability and Cognition: The Acquisition of Argument Structure. Cambridge MA: MIT Press.

Plaut, D.C. (1996). Relearning after damage in connectionist networks: toward a theory of rehabilitation. Brain and Language, 52, 25–82.

Plaut, D. and Shallice, T. (1993). Deep dyslexia: a case study of connectionist neuropsychology. Cognitive Neuropsychology, 10, 377–500.

Pound, C. (1996). Pound steady as City banks on change. Bulletin of the College of Speech and Language Therapists, Issue 532.

Pring, T., White-Thomson, M., Pound, C., Marshall, J. and Davis, A. (1990). Picture/word matching tasks and word retrieval: some follow-up data and second thoughts. Aphasiology, 4, 479–83.

Prizant, B.M. and Schuler, A.L. (1987). Facilitating communication: theoretical foundations. In D.J. Cohen, A.M. Donellan and R. Paul (eds.), Handbook of Autism and Pervasive Developmental Disorders. London: Wiley.

Rapin, I. (1987). Developmental dysphasia and autism in pre-school children: characteristics and sub-types. In Proceedings of the First International Symposium on Specific Speech and Language Disorders in Children. London: AFASIC.

Rapin, I. and Allen, D. (1983). Developmental language disorders: nosologic considerations. In U. Kirk (eds.), Neuropsychology of Language, Reading and Spelling. New York: Academic Press.

Rapin, I., Mattis, S., Rowan, A.J. and Golden, G.G. (1977). Verbal auditory agnosia in children. Developmental Medicine and Child Neurology, 19, 192–207.

Reilly, R.G. and Sharkey, N.E. (eds.). (1992). Connectionist Approaches to Natural Language Processing. Hove, Sussex: Erlbaum.

Reynell, J. and Huntley, M. (1985). The Reynell Developmental Language Scales Windsor: NFER NELSON.

Rice, M. and Bode, J. (1993). GAPS in the verb lexicon of children with specific language impairment. First Language, 13, 113–31.

Riddoch, M. and Humphreys, J. (1994). Cognitive Neuropsychology and Cognitive Rehabiliation. Hove, Sussex: Erlbaum.

Robertson, I., Tegner, R., Tham, K., Lo, A. and Nimmo-Smith, I. (1995). Sustained attention training for unilateral neglect: theoretical and rehabilitation implications. Journal of Clinical and Experimental Neuropsychology, 17, 416–30.

Ross, E. and Mesulam, M. (1979). Dominant language functions of the right hemisphere? Prosody and emotional gesturing. Archives of Neurology, 36, 561–9.

Roth, F. and Spekman, N. (1986). Narrative discourse: spontaneously generated stories of learning-disabled and normally achieving students. Journal of Speech and Hearing Disorders, 51, 8–23.

Rumelhart, D. (1980). Schemata: the building blocks of cognition. In R. Spiro, B. Bruce and W. Brewer (eds.), Theoretical Issues in Reading Comprehension: Perspectives from Cognitive Psychology, Linguistics, AI and Education. Hillsdale, NJ: Erlbaum.

Rumelhart, D. and McClelland, J. (eds.), (1986). Parallel Distributed Processing: Explorations in the Microstructure of Cognition. Cambridge, MA: MIT Press.

Rust, J., Golombok, S. and Trickey, G. (1993). Wechsler Objective Reading Dimensions. New York: Psychological Corporation.

Sacchett, C. and Humphreys, G. (1992). Calling a squirrel a squirrel but a canoe a wig-wam. A category specific deficit for artefactual objects and body parts. Cognitive Neuropsychology, 9, 73–86.

Sacks, O. (1985). The Man who Mistook his Wife for a Hat. London: Duckworth.

Saffran, E., Schwartz, M. and Marin, O. (1980). Evidence from aphasia: isolating the components of a production model. In B. Butterworth (eds.), Language Production. London: Academic Press.

Schegloff, E.A. and Sacks, H. (1973). Openings and closings. Semiotica, 7, 289–327.

Schuell, H. (1953). Aphasic difficulties understanding spoken language. Neurology, 3, 176–84.

Schwartz, E., Saffran, E., Fink, R., Myers, J. and Martin, N. (1994). Mapping therapy: a treatment programme for agrammatism. Aphasiology, 8, 19–54.

Schwartz, M., Linebarger, M., Saffran, E. and Pate, D. (1987). Syntactic transparency and sentence interpretation in aphasia. Language and Cognitive Processes, 2, 85–113.

Scott, C. (1987). Cognitive neuropsychological remediation of acquired language disorders. Unpublished MPhil thesis, Birkbeck College, University of London.

Semel, E., Wiig, E.H. and Secord, W. (1980). Clinical Evaluation of Language Fundamentals (revised). New York: Psychological Corporation.

Shallice, T. (1988). From Neuropsychology to Mental Structure. Cambridge: Cambridge University Press.

Sharkey, N.E. and Sharkey, A.J.C. (1990). Final Report to Leverhulme Trust: 'Learning Novel Words in Context'. Grant Ref No A/87/153;S/87/2693; F.213H.

Sherratt, S. and Penn, C. (1990). Discourse in a right-hemisphere brain-damaged subject. Aphasiology, 4, 539–60.

Sheridan, J. and Humphreys, G. (1993). A verbal-semantic category-specific recognition impairment. Cognitive Neuropsychology, 10, 143–84.

Shields, J., Varley, R., Broks, P. and Simpson, A. (1996). Hemispheric function in developmental language disorders and high-level autism. Developmental Medicine and Child Neurology, 38, 473–86.

Speake, J. and Bigland-Lewis, S. (1995). Semantic Connections. Ponteland: STASS Publications.

Spencer, A. (1988). A phonological theory of phonological development. In M.J. Ball (eds.), Theoretical linguistics and disordered language. London: Croom Helm.

Sperber, D. and Wilson, D. (1986). Relevance: Communication and Cognition. Oxford: Blackwell.

Spreen, O. and Benton, A.L. (1969). Neurosensory Center Comprehensive Examination for Aphasia. Victoria: University of Victoria.

Stackhouse, J. and Wells, B. (1993). Psycholinguistic assessment of developmental speech disorders. European Journal of Disorders of Communication, 28, 331–48.

Stackhouse, J. and Wells, B. (forthcoming). Psycholinguistic Assessment of Children with Speech and Literacy Difficulties. London: Whurr.

Stefanatos, G.A. (1991). Landau-Kleffner syndrome: diagnosis and treatment (letter). Autism Research Review International, 5, 6.

Stephanie, L. (1993). Letterland. Leatherhead: Letterland Direct.

Stroop, J. (1935). Studies in interference in serial verbal reactions. Journal of Experimental Psychology, 18, 643–62.

Stubbs, M. (1983). Discourse Analysis. Oxford: Blackwell.

Suzuki, S. and Notoya, M. (1980). Language therapy in pure word deafness in children: a case report. Auris Nasus Larynx, 7, 89–96.

Tager-Flusberg, H. (1981). On the nature of linguistic functioning in early infantile autism. Journal of Autism and Developmental Disorders, 11, 45–56.

Tallal, P. and Piercy, M. (1973). Developmental aphasia: impaired rate of non-verbal processing as a function of sensory modality. Neuropsychologia, 11, 389–98.

Tanenhaus, M. (1988). Psycholinguistics: an overview. In F. Newmeyer (eds.), Linguistics: The Cambridge Survey, Vol.4, pp. 1–37. Cambridge: Cambridge University Press.

Tönkovich, J. (1989). Managing pragmatic communication deficits associated with right hemisphere damage. Seminars in Speech and Language, 10, 343–54.

Trueswell, J.C., Tanenhaus, M.K. and Garnsey, S.M. (1994). Semantic influences on parsing: use of thematic role information in syntactic ambiguity resolution. Journal of Memory and Language, 33, 285–318.

Tyler, L.K. (1992). Spoken Language Comprehension: An Experimental Approach to Disordered and Normal Processing. Cambridge, MA: MIT Press.

Van de Lely, H. (1993). Specific language impairment in children: research findings and their therapeutic implications. European Journal of Disorders of Communication, 28, 247–63.

Vance, M. (1991). Educational and therapeutic approaches used with a child presenting with acquired aphasia with convulsive disorder (Landau-Kleffner syndrome). Child Language, Teaching and Therapy, 7, 41–60.

Vance, M. (1996). Assessing speech processing skills in children: a task analysis. In M. Snowling and J. Stackhouse (eds.), Dyslexia, Speech and Language: A Practitioner's Handbook. London:Whurr.

Varley, R. (1991). Reference, sense and antonymy in the assessment of lexical semantic abilities in aphasia. Aphasiology, 5, 149–70.

Varley, R. (1995). Lexical-semantic deficits following right hemisphere damage: evidence from verbal fluency tasks. European Journal of Disorders of Communication, 30, 362–71.

Warrington, E. and Shallice, T. (1984). Category specific semantic impairments. Brain, 107, 929–54.

Wechsler, D. (1992). Wechsler Intelligence Scales for Children III – UK. New York: Kent Psychological Corporation.

Wilkinson, R. (1995). Aphasia: conversation analysis of a non-fluent aphasic person. In M. Perkins and S. Howard (eds.), Case Studies in Clinical Linguistics. London: Whurr.

Willcox, A.H.E. and Mogford-Bevan, K. (1995a). Assessing conversational disability. Clinical Linguistics and Phonetics 9, 235–54.

Willcox, A.H.E. and Mogford-Bevan, K. (1995b). Conversational disability: assessment and remediation. In M. Perkins and S. Howard (eds.), Case Studies in Clinical Linguistics. London: Whurr.

Wimmer, H. and Perner, J. (1983). Beliefs about beliefs: representation and the constraining function of wrong belief in young children's understanding of deception. Cognition, 13, 103–28.

Winner, E. and Gardner, H. (1977). The comprehension of metaphor in brain damaged patients. Brain, 100, 719–27.

Worster-Drought, C. (1971). An unusual form of acquired aphasia in children. Developmental Medicine and Child Neurology, 13, 563–71.

Young, A. and Ratcliffe, G. (1983). Visuospatial abilities of the right hemisphere. In A.W. Yound (eds.), Functions of the Right Cerebral Hemisphere. London: Academic Press.

Index